Mometrix
TEST PREPARATION

AF901374

P-NAT

Secrets Study Guide

DEAR FUTURE EXAM SUCCESS STORY

First of all, **THANK YOU** for purchasing Mometrix study materials!

Second, congratulations! You are one of the few determined test-takers who are committed to doing whatever it takes to excel on your exam. **You have come to the right place.** We developed these study materials with one goal in mind: to deliver you the information you need in a format that's concise and easy to use.

In addition to optimizing your guide for the content of the test, we've outlined our recommended steps for breaking down the preparation process into small, attainable goals so you can make sure you stay on track.

We've also analyzed the entire test-taking process, identifying the most common pitfalls and showing how you can overcome them and be ready for any curveball the test throws you.

Standardized testing is one of the biggest obstacles on your road to success, which only increases the importance of doing well in the high-pressure, high-stakes environment of test day. Your results on this test could have a significant impact on your future, and this guide provides the information and practical advice to help you achieve your full potential on test day.

Your success is our success

We would love to hear from you! If you would like to share the story of your exam success or if you have any questions or comments in regard to our products, please contact us at **800-673-8175** or **support@mometrix.com**.

Thanks again for your business and we wish you continued success!

Sincerely,
The Mometrix Test Preparation Team

Need more help? Check out our flashcards at:
http://MometrixFlashcards.com/PNAT

Written and edited by the Mometrix Exam Secrets Test Prep Team
Printed in the United States of America

TABLE OF CONTENTS

INTRODUCTION 1
SECRET KEY 1: PLAN BIG, STUDY SMALL 2
SECRET KEY #2 – MAKE YOUR STUDYING COUNT 3
SECRET KEY 3: PRACTICE THE RIGHT WAY 4
SECRET KEY 4: PACE YOURSELF 6
SECRET KEY 5: HAVE A PLAN FOR GUESSING 7
TEST-TAKING STRATEGIES 10
READING COMPREHENSION AND REASONING ABILITY 15
WORD ROOTS AND PREFIXES AND SUFFIXES 15
NUANCE AND WORD MEANINGS 18
USING CONTEXT TO DETERMINE MEANING 20
RESOURCES FOR DETERMINING WORD MEANING AND USAGE 23
MAIN IDEAS AND SUPPORTING DETAILS 24
AUTHOR'S PURPOSE 25
COMMON ORGANIZATIONS OF TEXTS 27
MAKING AND EVALUATING PREDICTIONS 30
MAKING INFERENCES AND DRAWING CONCLUSIONS 31
CRITICAL READING SKILLS 32
PERSUASION AND RHETORIC 33
READING INFORMATIONAL TEXTS 35
ORGANIZATIONAL FEATURES IN TEXTS 37
TECHNICAL LANGUAGE 38
TYPES OF TECHNICAL WRITING 39
VISUAL INFORMATION IN INFORMATIONAL TEXTS 40
READING ARGUMENTATIVE WRITING 43
PLOT AND STORY STRUCTURE 45
NARRATOR'S POINT OF VIEW 48
SETTING, MOOD, AND TONE 50
CHARACTER DEVELOPMENT AND DIALOGUE 52
FIGURATIVE LANGUAGE 53
LITERARY DEVICES 57
CHAPTER QUIZ 58
NUMERICAL ABILITY 59
NUMBER BASICS 59
NUMBER LINES 60
COMPARING NUMBERS 61
ROUNDING AND ESTIMATION 62
ABSOLUTE VALUE 62
OPERATIONS 63
SUBTRACTION WITH REGROUPING 65
ORDER OF OPERATIONS 66

Properties of Operations 67
Properties of Exponents 69
Scientific Notation 69
Factors and Multiples 70
Fractions 71
Decimals 74
Percentages 75
Converting Between Percentages, Fractions, and Decimals 77
Rational and Irrational Numbers 78
Proportions and Ratios 78
Chapter Quiz 80

Language Ability 81
Parts of Speech 81
Agreement and Sentence Structure 90
Punctuation 107
Common Usage Mistakes 113
Spelling Conventions 118
Chapter Quiz 123

P-NAT Practice Test 124

Answer Key and Explanations 150

How to Overcome Test Anxiety 162

Online Resources 168

Introduction

Thank you for purchasing this resource! You have made the choice to prepare yourself for a test that could have a huge impact on your future, and this guide is designed to help you be fully ready for test day. Obviously, it's important to have a solid understanding of the test material, but you also need to be prepared for the unique environment and stressors of the test, so that you can perform to the best of your abilities.

For this purpose, the first section that appears in this guide is the **Secret Keys**. We've devoted countless hours to meticulously researching what works and what doesn't, and we've boiled down our findings to the five most impactful steps you can take to improve your performance on the test. We start at the beginning with study planning and move through the preparation process, all the way to the testing strategies that will help you get the most out of what you know when you're finally sitting in front of the test.

We recommend that you start preparing for your test as far in advance as possible. However, if you've bought this guide as a last-minute study resource and only have a few days before your test, we recommend that you skip over the first two Secret Keys since they address a long-term study plan.

If you struggle with **test anxiety**, we strongly encourage you to check out our recommendations for how you can overcome it. Test anxiety is a formidable foe, but it can be beaten, and we want to make sure you have the tools you need to defeat it.

Secret Key 1: Plan Big, Study Small

There's a lot riding on your performance. If you want to ace this test, you're going to need to keep your skills sharp and the material fresh in your mind. You need a plan that lets you review everything you need to know while still fitting in your schedule. We'll break this strategy down into three categories.

Information Organization

Start with the information you already have: the official test outline. From this, you can make a complete list of all the concepts you need to cover before the test. Organize these concepts into groups that can be studied together, and create a list of any related vocabulary you need to learn so you can brush up on any difficult terms. You'll want to keep this vocabulary list handy once you actually start studying since you may need to add to it along the way.

Time Management

Once you have your set of study concepts, decide how to spread them out over the time you have left before the test. Break your study plan into small, clear goals so you have a manageable task for each day and know exactly what you're doing. Then just focus on one small step at a time. When you manage your time this way, you don't need to spend hours at a time studying. Studying a small block of content for a short period each day helps you retain information better and avoid stressing over how much you have left to do. You can relax knowing that you have a plan to cover everything in time. In order for this strategy to be effective though, you have to start studying early and stick to your schedule. Avoid the exhaustion and futility that comes from last-minute cramming!

Study Environment

The environment you study in has a big impact on your learning. Studying in a coffee shop, while probably more enjoyable, is not likely to be as fruitful as studying in a quiet room. It's important to keep distractions to a minimum. You're only planning to study for a short block of time, so make the most of it. Don't pause to check your phone or get up to find a snack. It's also important to **avoid multitasking**. Research has consistently shown that multitasking will make your studying dramatically less effective. Your study area should also be comfortable and well-lit so you don't have the distraction of straining your eyes or sitting on an uncomfortable chair.

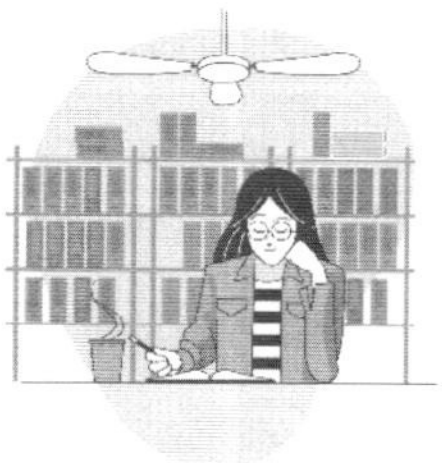

The time of day you study is also important. You want to be rested and alert. Don't wait until just before bedtime. Study when you'll be most likely to comprehend and remember. Even better, if you know what time of day your test will be, set that time aside for study. That way your brain will be used to working on that subject at that specific time and you'll have a better chance of recalling information.

Finally, it can be helpful to team up with others who are studying for the same test. Your actual studying should be done in as isolated an environment as possible, but the work of organizing the information and setting up the study plan can be divided up. In between study sessions, you can discuss with your teammates the concepts that you're all studying and quiz each other on the details. Just be sure that your teammates are as serious about the test as you are. If you find that your study time is being replaced with social time, you might need to find a new team.

Secret Key #2 – Make Your Studying Count

You're devoting a lot of time and effort to preparing for this test, so you want to be absolutely certain it will pay off. This means doing more than just reading the content and hoping you can remember it on test day. It's important to make every minute of study count. There are two main areas you can focus on to make your studying count.

Retention

It doesn't matter how much time you study if you can't remember the material. You need to make sure you are retaining the concepts. To check your retention of the information you're learning, try recalling it at later times with minimal prompting. Try carrying around flashcards and glance at one or two from time to time or ask a friend who's also studying for the test to quiz you.

To enhance your retention, look for ways to put the information into practice so that you can apply it rather than simply recalling it. If you're using the information in practical ways, it will be much easier to remember. Similarly, it helps to solidify a concept in your mind if you're not only reading it to yourself but also explaining it to someone else. Ask a friend to let you teach them about a concept you're a little shaky on (or speak aloud to an imaginary audience if necessary). As you try to summarize, define, give examples, and answer your friend's questions, you'll understand the concepts better and they will stay with you longer. Finally, step back for a big picture view and ask yourself how each piece of information fits with the whole subject. When you link the different concepts together and see them working together as a whole, it's easier to remember the individual components.

Finally, practice showing your work on any multi-step problems, even if you're just studying. Writing out each step you take to solve a problem will help solidify the process in your mind, and you'll be more likely to remember it during the test.

Modality

Modality simply refers to the means or method by which you study. Choosing a study modality that fits your own individual learning style is crucial. No two people learn best in exactly the same way, so it's important to know your strengths and use them to your advantage.

For example, if you learn best by visualization, focus on visualizing a concept in your mind and draw an image or a diagram. Try color-coding your notes, illustrating them, or creating symbols that will trigger your mind to recall a learned concept. If you learn best by hearing or discussing information, find a study partner who learns the same way or read aloud to yourself. Think about how to put the information in your own words. Imagine that you are giving a lecture on the topic and record yourself so you can listen to it later.

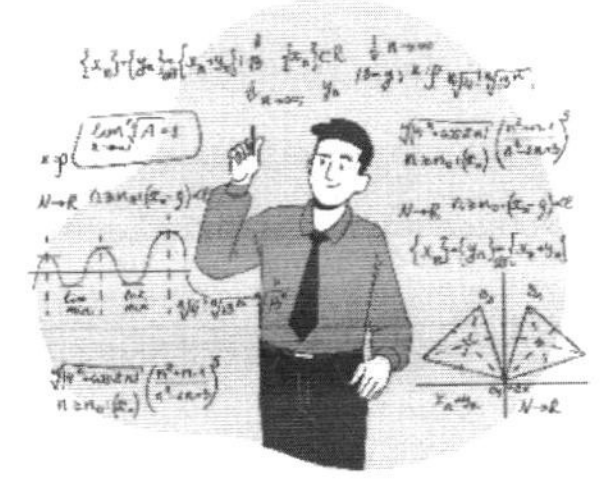

For any learning style, flashcards can be helpful. Organize the information so you can take advantage of spare moments to review. Underline key words or phrases. Use different colors for different categories. Mnemonic devices (such as creating a short list in which every item starts with the same letter) can also help with retention. Find what works best for you and use it to store the information in your mind most effectively and easily.

Secret Key 3: Practice the Right Way

Your success on test day depends not only on how many hours you put into preparing, but also on whether you prepared the right way. It's good to check along the way to see if your studying is paying off. One of the most effective ways to do this is by taking practice tests to evaluate your progress. Practice tests are useful because they show exactly where you need to improve. Every time you take a practice test, pay special attention to these three groups of questions:

- The questions you got wrong
- The questions you had to guess on, even if you guessed right
- The questions you found difficult or slow to work through

This will show you exactly what your weak areas are, and where you need to devote more study time. Ask yourself why each of these questions gave you trouble. Was it because you didn't understand the material? Was it because you didn't remember the vocabulary? Do you need more repetitions on this type of question to build speed and confidence? Dig into those questions and figure out how you can strengthen your weak areas as you go back to review the material.

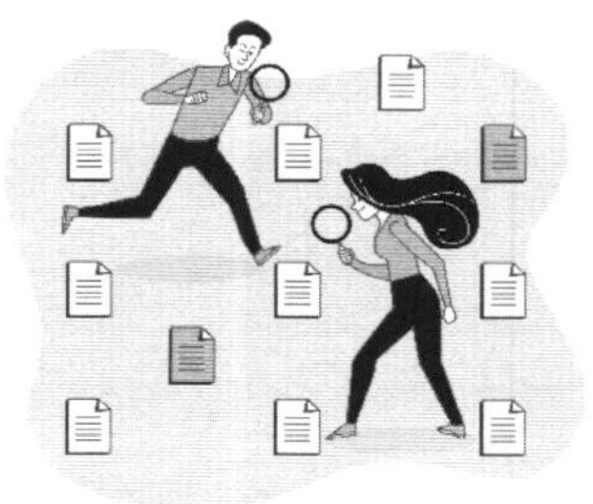

Additionally, many practice tests have a section explaining the answer choices. It can be tempting to read the explanation and think that you now have a good understanding of the concept. However, an explanation likely only covers part of the question's broader context. Even if the explanation makes perfect sense, **go back and investigate** every concept related to the question until you're positive you have a thorough understanding.

As you go along, keep in mind that the practice test is just that: practice. Memorizing these questions and answers will not be very helpful on the actual test because it is unlikely to have any of the same exact questions. If you only know the right answers to the sample questions, you won't be prepared for the real thing. **Study the concepts** until you understand them fully, and then you'll be able to answer any question that shows up on the test.

It's important to wait on the practice tests until you're ready. If you take a test on your first day of study, you may be overwhelmed by the amount of material covered and how much you need to learn. Work up to it gradually.

On test day, you'll need to be prepared for answering questions, managing your time, and using the test-taking strategies you've learned. It's a lot to balance, like a mental marathon that will have a big impact on your future. Like training for a marathon, you'll need to start slowly and work your way up. When test day arrives, you'll be ready.

Start with the strategies you've read in the first two Secret Keys—plan your course and study in the way that works best for you. If you have time, consider using multiple study resources to get different approaches to the same concepts. It can be helpful to see difficult concepts from more than one angle. Then find a good source for practice tests. Many times, the test website will suggest potential study resources or provide sample tests.

Practice Test Strategy

If you're able to find at least three practice tests, we recommend this strategy:

Untimed and Open-Book Practice

Take the first test with no time constraints and with your notes and study guide handy. Take your time and focus on applying the strategies you've learned.

Timed and Open-Book Practice

Take the second practice test open-book as well, but set a timer and practice pacing yourself to finish in time.

Timed and Closed-Book Practice

Take any other practice tests as if it were test day. Set a timer and put away your study materials. Sit at a table or desk in a quiet room, imagine yourself at the testing center, and answer questions as quickly and accurately as possible.

Keep repeating timed and closed-book tests on a regular basis until you run out of practice tests or it's time for the actual test. Your mind will be ready for the schedule and stress of test day, and you'll be able to focus on recalling the material you've learned.

Secret Key 4: Pace Yourself

Once you're fully prepared for the material on the test, your biggest challenge on test day will be managing your time. Just knowing that the clock is ticking can make you panic even if you have plenty of time left. Work on pacing yourself so you can build confidence against the time constraints of the exam. Pacing is a difficult skill to master, especially in a high-pressure environment, so **practice is vital**.

Set time expectations for your pace based on how much time is available. For example, if a section has 60 questions and the time limit is 30 minutes, you know you have to average 30 seconds or less per question in order to answer them all. Although 30 seconds is the hard limit, set 25 seconds per question as your goal, so you reserve extra time to spend on harder questions. When you budget extra time for the harder questions, you no longer have any reason to stress when those questions take longer to answer.

Don't let this time expectation distract you from working through the test at a calm, steady pace, but keep it in mind so you don't spend too much time on any one question. Recognize that taking extra time on one question you don't understand may keep you from answering two that you do understand later in the test. If your time limit for a question is up and you're still not sure of the answer, mark it and move on, and come back to it later if the time and the test format allow. If the testing format doesn't allow you to return to earlier questions, just make an educated guess; then put it out of your mind and move on.

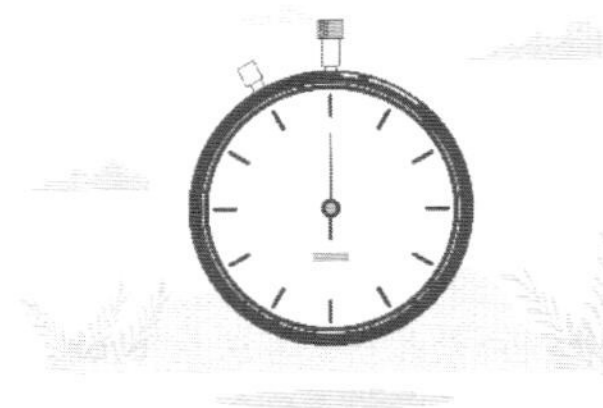

On the easier questions, be careful not to rush. It may seem wise to hurry through them so you have more time for the challenging ones, but it's not worth missing one if you know the concept and just didn't take the time to read the question fully. Work efficiently but make sure you understand the question and have looked at all of the answer choices, since more than one may seem right at first.

Even if you're paying attention to the time, you may find yourself a little behind at some point. You should speed up to get back on track, but do so wisely. Don't panic; just take a few seconds less on each question until you're caught up. Don't guess without thinking, but do look through the answer choices and eliminate any you know are wrong. If you can get down to two choices, it is often worthwhile to guess from those. Once you've chosen an answer, move on and don't dwell on any that you skipped or had to hurry through. If a question was taking too long, chances are it was one of the harder ones, so you weren't as likely to get it right anyway.

On the other hand, if you find yourself getting ahead of schedule, it may be beneficial to slow down a little. The more quickly you work, the more likely you are to make a careless mistake that will affect your score. You've budgeted time for each question, so don't be afraid to spend that time. Practice an efficient but careful pace to get the most out of the time you have.

Secret Key 5: Have a Plan for Guessing

When you're taking the test, you may find yourself stuck on a question. Some of the answer choices seem better than others, but you don't see the one answer choice that is obviously correct. What do you do?

The scenario described above is very common, yet most test takers have not effectively prepared for it. Developing and practicing a plan for guessing may be one of the single most effective uses of your time as you get ready for the exam.

In developing your plan for guessing, there are three questions to address:

- When should you start the guessing process?
- How should you narrow down the choices?
- Which answer should you choose?

When to Start the Guessing Process

Unless your plan for guessing is to select C every time (which, despite its merits, is not what we recommend), you need to leave yourself enough time to apply your answer elimination strategies. Since you have a limited amount of time for each question, that means that if you're going to give yourself the best shot at guessing correctly, you have to decide quickly whether or not you will guess.

Of course, the best-case scenario is that you don't have to guess at all, so first, see if you can answer the question based on your knowledge of the subject and basic reasoning skills. Focus on the key words in the question and try to jog your memory of related topics. Give yourself a chance to bring the knowledge to mind, but once you realize that you don't have (or you can't access) the knowledge you need to answer the question, it's time to start the guessing process.

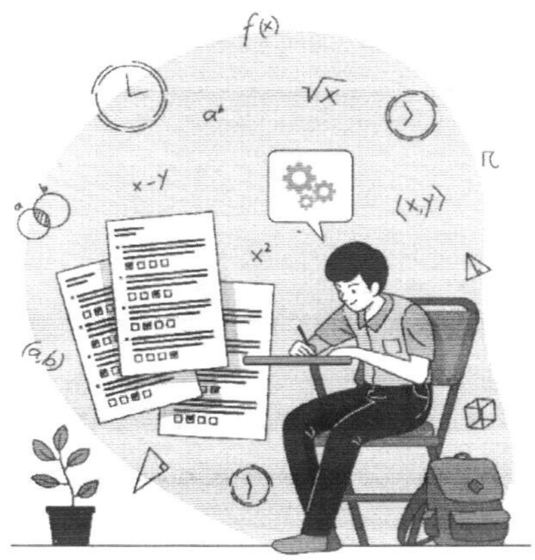

It's almost always better to start the guessing process too early than too late. It only takes a few seconds to remember something and answer the question from knowledge. Carefully eliminating wrong answer choices takes longer. Plus, going through the process of eliminating answer choices can actually help jog your memory.

Summary: Start the guessing process as soon as you decide that you can't answer the question based on your knowledge.

How to Narrow Down the Choices

The next chapter in this book (**Test-Taking Strategies**) includes a wide range of strategies for how to approach questions and how to look for answer choices to eliminate. You will definitely want to read those carefully, practice them, and figure out which ones work best for you. Here though, we're going to address a mindset rather than a particular strategy.

Your odds of guessing an answer correctly depend on how many options you are choosing from.

Number of options left	5	4	3	2	1
Odds of guessing correctly	20%	25%	33%	50%	100%

You can see from this chart just how valuable it is to be able to eliminate incorrect answers and make an educated guess, but there are two things that many test takers do that cause them to miss out on the benefits of guessing:

- Accidentally eliminating the correct answer
- Selecting an answer based on an impression

We'll look at the first one here, and the second one in the next section.

To avoid accidentally eliminating the correct answer, we recommend a thought exercise called **the $5 challenge**. In this challenge, you only eliminate an answer choice from contention if you are willing to bet $5 on it being wrong. Why $5? Five dollars is a small but not insignificant amount of money. It's an amount you could afford to lose but wouldn't want to throw away. And while losing $5 once might not hurt too much, doing it twenty times will set you back $100. In the same way, each small decision you make—eliminating a choice here, guessing on a question there—won't by itself impact your score very much, but when you put them all together, they can make a big difference. By holding each answer choice elimination decision to a higher standard, you can reduce the risk of accidentally eliminating the correct answer.

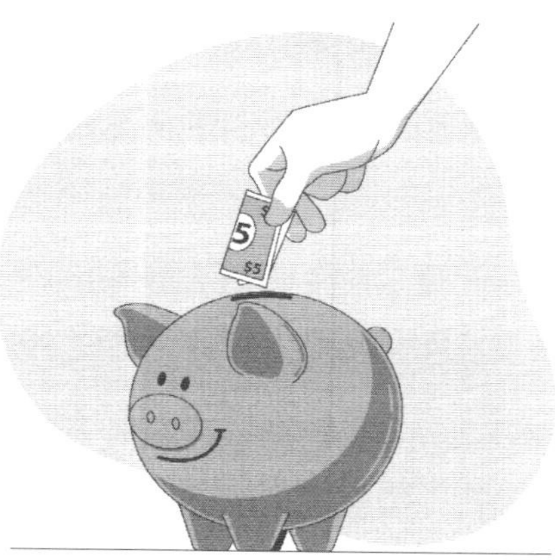

The $5 challenge can also be applied in a positive sense: If you are willing to bet $5 that an answer choice *is* correct, go ahead and mark it as correct.

Summary: Only eliminate an answer choice if you are willing to bet $5 that it is wrong.

Which Answer to Choose

You're taking the test. You've run into a hard question and decided you'll have to guess. You've eliminated all the answer choices you're willing to bet $5 on. Now you have to pick an answer. Why do we even need to talk about this? Why can't you just pick whichever one you feel like when the time comes?

The answer to these questions is that if you don't come into the test with a plan, you'll rely on your impression to select an answer choice, and if you do that, you risk falling into a trap. The test writers know that everyone who takes their test will be guessing on some of the questions, so they intentionally write wrong answer choices to seem plausible. You still have to pick an answer though, and if the wrong answer choices are designed to look right, how can you ever be sure that you're not falling for their trap? The best solution we've found to this dilemma is to take the decision out of your hands entirely. Here is the process we recommend:

Once you've eliminated any choices that you are confident (willing to bet $5) are wrong, select the first remaining choice as your answer.

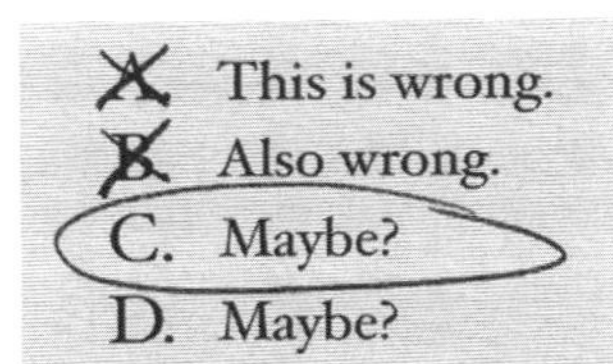

Whether you choose to select the first remaining choice, the second, or the last, the important thing is that you use some preselected standard. Using this approach guarantees that you will not be enticed into selecting an answer choice that looks right, because you are not basing your decision on how the answer choices look.

This is not meant to make you question your knowledge. Instead, it is to help you recognize the difference between your knowledge and your impressions. There's a huge difference between thinking an answer is right because of what you know, and thinking an answer is right because it looks or sounds like it should be right.

Summary: To ensure that your selection is appropriately random, make a predetermined selection from among all answer choices you have not eliminated.

Test-Taking Strategies

This section contains a list of test-taking strategies that you may find helpful as you work through the test. By taking what you know and applying logical thought, you can maximize your chances of answering any question correctly!

It is very important to realize that every question is different and every person is different: no single strategy will work on every question, and no single strategy will work for every person. That's why we've included all of them here, so you can try them out and determine which ones work best for different types of questions and which ones work best for you.

Question Strategies

✓ Read Carefully

Read the question and the answer choices carefully. Don't miss the question because you misread the terms. You have plenty of time to read each question thoroughly and make sure you understand what is being asked. Yet a happy medium must be attained, so don't waste too much time. You must read carefully and efficiently.

✓ Contextual Clues

Look for contextual clues. If the question includes a word you are not familiar with, look at the immediate context for some indication of what the word might mean. Contextual clues can often give you all the information you need to decipher the meaning of an unfamiliar word. Even if you can't determine the meaning, you may be able to narrow down the possibilities enough to make a solid guess at the answer to the question.

✓ Prefixes

If you're having trouble with a word in the question or answer choices, try dissecting it. Take advantage of every clue that the word might include. Prefixes can be a huge help. Usually, they allow you to determine a basic meaning. *Pre-* means before, *post-* means after, *pro-* is positive, *de-* is negative. From prefixes, you can get an idea of the general meaning of the word and try to put it into context.

✓ Hedge Words

Watch out for critical hedge words, such as *likely, may, can, often, almost, mostly, usually, generally, rarely*, and *sometimes*. Question writers insert these hedge phrases to cover every possibility. Often an answer choice will be wrong simply because it leaves no room for exception. Be on guard for answer choices that have definitive words such as *exactly* and *always*.

✓ Switchback Words

Stay alert for *switchbacks*. These are the words and phrases frequently used to alert you to shifts in thought. The most common switchback words are *but, although*, and *however*. Others include *nevertheless, on the other hand, even though, while, in spite of, despite*, and *regardless of*. Switchback words are important to catch because they can change the direction of the question or an answer choice.

✓ Face Value

When in doubt, use common sense. Accept the situation in the problem at face value. Don't read too much into it. These problems will not require you to make wild assumptions. If you have to go beyond creativity and warp time or space in order to have an answer choice fit the question, then you should move on and consider the other answer choices. These are normal problems rooted in reality. The applicable relationship or explanation may not be readily apparent, but it is there for you to figure out. Use your common sense to interpret anything that isn't clear.

Answer Choice Strategies

✓ Answer Selection

The most thorough way to pick an answer choice is to identify and eliminate wrong answers until only one is left, then confirm it is the correct answer. Sometimes an answer choice may immediately seem right, but be careful. The test writers will usually put more than one reasonable answer choice on each question, so take a second to read all of them and make sure that the other choices are not equally obvious. As long as you have time left, it is better to read every answer choice than to pick the first one that looks right without checking the others.

✓ Answer Choice Families

An answer choice family consists of two (in rare cases, three) answer choices that are very similar in construction and cannot all be true at the same time. If you see two answer choices that are direct opposites or parallels, one of them is usually the correct answer. For instance, if one answer choice says that quantity *x* increases and another either says that quantity *x* decreases (opposite) or says that quantity *y* increases (parallel), then those answer choices would fall into the same family. An answer choice that doesn't match the construction of the answer choice family is more likely to be incorrect. Most questions will not have answer choice families, but when they do appear, you should be prepared to recognize them.

✓ Eliminate Answers

Eliminate answer choices as soon as you realize they are wrong, but make sure you consider all possibilities. If you are eliminating answer choices and realize that the last one you are left with is also wrong, don't panic. Start over and consider each choice again. There may be something you missed the first time that you will realize on the second pass.

✓ Avoid Fact Traps

Don't be distracted by an answer choice that is factually true but doesn't answer the question. You are looking for the choice that answers the question. Stay focused on what the question is asking for so you don't accidentally pick an answer that is true but incorrect. Always go back to the question and make sure the answer choice you've selected actually answers the question and is not merely a true statement.

✓ Extreme Statements

In general, you should avoid answers that put forth extreme actions as standard practice or proclaim controversial ideas as established fact. An answer choice that states the "process should be used in certain situations, if..." is much more likely to be correct than one that states the "process should be discontinued completely." The first is a calm rational statement and doesn't even make a definitive, uncompromising stance, using a hedge word *if* to provide wiggle room, whereas the second choice is far more extreme.

⊘ Benchmark

As you read through the answer choices and you come across one that seems to answer the question well, mentally select that answer choice. This is not your final answer, but it's the one that will help you evaluate the other answer choices. The one that you selected is your benchmark or standard for judging each of the other answer choices. Every other answer choice must be compared to your benchmark. That choice is correct until proven otherwise by another answer choice beating it. If you find a better answer, then that one becomes your new benchmark. Once you've decided that no other choice answers the question as well as your benchmark, you have your final answer.

⊘ Predict the Answer

Before you even start looking at the answer choices, it is often best to try to predict the answer. When you come up with the answer on your own, it is easier to avoid distractions and traps because you will know exactly what to look for. The right answer choice is unlikely to be word-for-word what you came up with, but it should be a close match. Even if you are confident that you have the right answer, you should still take the time to read each option before moving on.

General Strategies

⊘ Tough Questions

If you are stumped on a problem or it appears too hard or too difficult, don't waste time. Move on! Remember though, if you can quickly check for obviously incorrect answer choices, your chances of guessing correctly are greatly improved. Before you completely give up, at least try to knock out a couple of possible answers. Eliminate what you can and then guess at the remaining answer choices before moving on.

⊘ Check Your Work

Since you will probably not know every term listed and the answer to every question, it is important that you get credit for the ones that you do know. Don't miss any questions through careless mistakes. If at all possible, try to take a second to look back over your answer selection and make sure you've selected the correct answer choice and haven't made a costly careless mistake (such as marking an answer choice that you didn't mean to mark). This quick double check should more than pay for itself in caught mistakes for the time it costs.

⊘ Pace Yourself

It's easy to be overwhelmed when you're looking at a page full of questions; your mind is confused and full of random thoughts, and the clock is ticking down faster than you would like. Calm down and maintain the pace that you have set for yourself. Especially as you get down to the last few minutes of the test, don't let the small numbers on the clock make you panic. As long as you are on track by monitoring your pace, you are guaranteed to have time for each question.

⊘ Don't Rush

It is very easy to make errors when you are in a hurry. Maintaining a fast pace in answering questions is pointless if it makes you miss questions that you would have gotten right otherwise. Test writers like to include distracting information and wrong answers that seem right. Taking a little extra time to avoid careless mistakes can make all the difference in your test score. Find a pace that allows you to be confident in the answers that you select.

⊘ KEEP MOVING

Panicking will not help you pass the test, so do your best to stay calm and keep moving. Taking deep breaths and going through the answer elimination steps you practiced can help to break through a stress barrier and keep your pace.

Final Notes

The combination of a solid foundation of content knowledge and the confidence that comes from practicing your plan for applying that knowledge is the key to maximizing your performance on test day. As your foundation of content knowledge is built up and strengthened, you'll find that the strategies included in this chapter become more and more effective in helping you quickly sift through the distractions and traps of the test to isolate the correct answer.

Now that you're preparing to move forward into the test content chapters of this book, be sure to keep your goal in mind. As you read, think about how you will be able to apply this information on the test. If you've already seen sample questions for the test and you have an idea of the question format and style, try to come up with questions of your own that you can answer based on what you're reading. This will give you valuable practice applying your knowledge in the same ways you can expect to on test day.

Good luck and good studying!

Reading Comprehension and Reasoning Ability

Word Roots and Prefixes and Suffixes

Affixes

Affixes in the English language are morphemes that are added to words to create related but different words. Derivational affixes form new words based on and related to the original words. For example, the affix *–ness* added to the end of the adjective *happy* forms the noun *happiness.* Inflectional affixes form different grammatical versions of words. For example, the plural affix *–s* changes the singular noun *book* to the plural noun *books*, and the past tense affix *–ed* changes the present tense verb *look* to the past tense *looked.* Prefixes are affixes placed in front of words. For example, *heat* means to make hot; *preheat* means to heat in advance. Suffixes are affixes placed at the ends of words. The *happiness* example above contains the suffix *–ness.* Circumfixes add parts both before and after words, such as how *light* becomes *enlighten* with the prefix *en-* and the suffix *–en.* Interfixes create compound words via central affixes: *speed* and *meter* become *speedometer* via the interfix *–o–*.

Review Video: Affixes
Visit mometrix.com/academy and enter code: 782422

Word Roots, Prefixes, and Suffixes to Help Determine Meanings of Words

Many English words were formed from combining multiple sources. For example, the Latin *habēre* means "to have," and the prefixes *in-* and *im-* mean a lack or prevention of something, as in *insufficient* and *imperfect.* Latin combined *in-* with *habēre* to form *inhibēre,* whose past participle was *inhibitus*. This is the origin of the English word *inhibit,* meaning to prevent from having. Hence by knowing the meanings of both the prefix and the root, one can decipher the word meaning. In Greek, the root *enkephalo-* refers to the brain. Many medical terms are based on this root, such as encephalitis and hydrocephalus. Understanding the prefix and suffix meanings (*-itis* means inflammation; *hydro-* means water) allows a person to deduce that encephalitis refers to brain inflammation and hydrocephalus refers to water (or other fluid) in the brain.

Review Video: Root Words in English
Visit mometrix.com/academy and enter code: 896380

Review Video: Determining Word Meanings
Visit mometrix.com/academy and enter code: 894894

Prefixes

Knowing common prefixes is helpful for all readers as they try to determining meanings or definitions of unfamiliar words. For example, a common word used when cooking is *preheat.* Knowing that *pre-* means in advance can also inform them that *presume* means to assume in advance, that *prejudice* means advance judgment, and that this understanding can be applied to many other words beginning with *pre-.* Knowing that the prefix *dis-* indicates opposition informs the meanings of words like *disbar, disagree, disestablish,* and many more. Knowing *dys-* means bad, impaired, abnormal, or difficult informs *dyslogistic, dysfunctional, dysphagia,* and *dysplasia.*

Suffixes

In English, certain suffixes generally indicate both that a word is a noun, and that the noun represents a state of being or quality. For example, *-ness* is commonly used to change an adjective into its noun form, as with *happy* and *happiness, nice* and *niceness,* and so on. The suffix *–tion* is commonly used to transform a verb into its noun form, as with *converse* and *conversation or move* and *motion*. Thus, if readers are unfamiliar with the second form of a word, knowing the meaning of the transforming suffix can help them determine meaning.

Prefixes for Numbers

Prefix	Definition	Examples
bi-	two	bisect, biennial
mono-	one, single	monogamy, monologue
poly-	many	polymorphous, polygamous
semi-	half, partly	semicircle, semicolon
uni-	one	uniform, unity

Prefixes for Time, Direction, and Space

Prefix	Definition	Examples
a-	in, on, of, up, to	abed, afoot
ab-	from, away, off	abdicate, abjure
ad-	to, toward	advance, adventure
ante-	before, previous	antecedent, antedate
anti-	against, opposing	antipathy, antidote
cata-	down, away, thoroughly	catastrophe, cataclysm
circum-	around	circumspect, circumference
com-	with, together, very	commotion, complicate
contra-	against, opposing	contradict, contravene
de-	from	depart
dia-	through, across, apart	diameter, diagnose
dis-	away, off, down, not	dissent, disappear
epi-	upon	epilogue
ex-	out	extract, excerpt
hypo-	under, beneath	hypodermic, hypothesis
inter-	among, between	intercede, interrupt
intra-	within	intramural, intrastate
ob-	against, opposing	objection
per-	through	perceive, permit
peri-	around	periscope, perimeter
post-	after, following	postpone, postscript
pre-	before, previous	prevent, preclude
pro-	forward, in place of	propel, pronoun
retro-	back, backward	retrospect, retrograde
sub-	under, beneath	subjugate, substitute
super-	above, extra	supersede, supernumerary
trans-	across, beyond, over	transact, transport
ultra-	beyond, excessively	ultramodern, ultrasonic

Negative Prefixes

Prefix	Definition	Examples
a-	without, lacking	atheist, agnostic
in-	not, opposing	incapable, ineligible
non-	not	nonentity, nonsense
un-	not, reverse of	unhappy, unlock

Extra Prefixes

Prefix	Definition	Examples
for-	away, off, from	forget, forswear
fore-	previous	foretell, forefathers
homo-	same, equal	homogenized, homonym
hyper-	excessive, over	hypercritical, hypertension
in-	in, into	intrude, invade
mal-	bad, poorly, not	malfunction, malpractice
mis-	bad, poorly, not	misspell, misfire
neo-	new	Neolithic, neoconservative
omni-	all, everywhere	omniscient, omnivore
ortho-	right, straight	orthogonal, orthodox
over-	above	overbearing, oversight
pan-	all, entire	panorama, pandemonium
para-	beside, beyond	parallel, paradox
re-	backward, again	revoke, recur
sym-	with, together	sympathy, symphony

Below is a list of common suffixes and their meanings:

Adjective Suffixes

Suffix	Definition	Examples
-able (-ible)	capable of being	toler*able*, ed*ible*
-esque	in the style of, like	picturesque, grotesque
-ful	filled with, marked by	thankful, zestful
-ific	make, cause	terrific, beatific
-ish	suggesting, like	churlish, childish
-less	lacking, without	hopeless, countless
-ous	marked by, given to	religious, riotous

Noun Suffixes

Suffix	Definition	Examples
-acy	state, condition	accuracy, privacy
-ance	act, condition, fact	acceptance, vigilance
-ard	one that does excessively	drunkard, sluggard
-ation	action, state, result	occupation, starvation
-dom	state, rank, condition	serfdom, wisdom
-er (-or)	office, action	teach*er*, elevat*or*, hon*or*
-ess	feminine	waitress, duchess
-hood	state, condition	manhood, statehood
-ion	action, result, state	union, fusion
-ism	act, manner, doctrine	barbarism, socialism

Suffix	Definition	Examples
-ist	worker, follower	monopolist, socialist
-ity (-ty)	state, quality, condition	acid*ity*, civil*ity*, twen*ty*
-ment	result, action	Refreshment
-ness	quality, state	greatness, tallness
-ship	position	internship, statesmanship
-sion (-tion)	state, result	revi*sion*, expedi*tion*
-th	act, state, quality	warmth, width
-tude	quality, state, result	magnitude, fortitude

VERB SUFFIXES

Suffix	Definition	Examples
-ate	having, showing	separate, desolate
-en	cause to be, become	deepen, strengthen
-fy	make, cause to have	glorify, fortify
-ize	cause to be, treat with	sterilize, mechanize

Nuance and Word Meanings

SYNONYMS AND ANTONYMS

When you understand how words relate to each other, you will discover more in a passage. This is explained by understanding **synonyms** (e.g., words that mean the same thing) and **antonyms** (e.g., words that mean the opposite of one another). As an example, *dry* and *arid* are synonyms, and *dry* and *wet* are antonyms.

There are many pairs of words in English that can be considered synonyms, despite having slightly different definitions. For instance, the words *friendly* and *collegial* can both be used to describe a warm interpersonal relationship, and one would be correct to call them synonyms. However, *collegial* (kin to *colleague*) is often used in reference to professional or academic relationships, and *friendly* has no such connotation.

If the difference between the two words is too great, then they should not be called synonyms. *Hot* and *warm* are not synonyms because their meanings are too distinct. A good way to determine whether two words are synonyms is to substitute one word for the other word and verify that the meaning of the sentence has not changed. Substituting *warm* for *hot* in a sentence would convey a different meaning. Although warm and hot may seem close in meaning, warm generally means that the temperature is moderate, and hot generally means that the temperature is excessively high.

Antonyms are words with opposite meanings. *Light* and *dark*, *up* and *down*, *right* and *left*, *good* and *bad*: these are all sets of antonyms. Be careful to distinguish between antonyms and pairs of words that are simply different. *Black* and *gray*, for instance, are not antonyms because gray is not the opposite of black. *Black* and *white*, on the other hand, are antonyms.

Not every word has an antonym. For instance, many nouns do not. What would be the antonym of *chair*? During your exam, the questions related to antonyms are more likely to concern adjectives. You will recall that adjectives are words that describe a noun. Some common adjectives include *purple, fast, skinny*, and *sweet*. From those four adjectives, *purple* is the item that lacks a group of obvious antonyms.

Review Video: Synonyms and Antonyms
Visit mometrix.com/academy and enter code: 105612

Denotative vs. Connotative Meaning

The **denotative** meaning of a word is the literal meaning. The **connotative** meaning goes beyond the denotative meaning to include the emotional reaction that a word may invoke. The connotative meaning often takes the denotative meaning a step further due to associations the reader makes with the denotative meaning. Readers can differentiate between the denotative and connotative meanings by first recognizing how authors use each meaning. Most non-fiction, for example, is fact-based and authors do not use flowery, figurative language. The reader can assume that the writer is using the denotative meaning of words. In fiction, the author may use the connotative meaning. Readers can determine whether the author is using the denotative or connotative meaning of a word by implementing context clues.

Review Video: Connotation and Denotation
Visit mometrix.com/academy and enter code: 310092

Nuances of Word Meaning

A word's denotation is simply its objective dictionary definition. However, its connotation refers to the subjective associations, often emotional, that specific words evoke in listeners and readers. Two or more words can have the same dictionary meaning, but very different connotations. Writers use diction (word choice) to convey various nuances of thought and emotion by selecting synonyms for other words that best communicate the associations they want to trigger for readers. For example, a car engine is naturally greasy; in this sense, "greasy" is a neutral term. But when a person's smile, appearance, or clothing is described as "greasy," it has a negative connotation. Some words have even gained additional or different meanings over time. For example, *awful* used to be used to describe things that evoked a sense of awe. When *awful* is separated into its root word, awe, and suffix, -ful, it can be understood to mean "full of awe." However, the word is now commonly used to describe things that evoke repulsion, terror, or another intense, negative reaction.

Review Video: Word Usage in Sentences
Visit mometrix.com/academy and enter code: 197863

Using Context to Determine Meaning

Context Clues

Readers of all levels will encounter words that they have either never seen or have encountered only on a limited basis. The best way to define a word in **context** is to look for nearby words that can assist in revealing the meaning of the word. For instance, unfamiliar nouns are often accompanied by examples that provide a definition. Consider the following sentence: *Dave arrived at the party in hilarious garb: a leopard-print shirt, buckskin trousers, and bright green sneakers.* If a reader was unfamiliar with the meaning of garb, he or she could read the examples (i.e., a leopard-print shirt, buckskin trousers, and bright green sneakers) and quickly determine that the word means *clothing*. Examples will not always be this obvious. Consider this sentence: *Parsley, lemon, and flowers were just a few of the items he used as garnishes.* Here, the word *garnishes* is exemplified by parsley, lemon, and flowers. Readers who have eaten in a variety of restaurants will probably be able to identify a garnish as something used to decorate a plate.

> **Review Video: Reading Comprehension: Using Context Clues**
> Visit mometrix.com/academy and enter code: 613660

Using Contrast in Context Clues

In addition to looking at the context of a passage, readers can use contrast to define an unfamiliar word in context. In many sentences, the author will not describe the unfamiliar word directly; instead, he or she will describe the opposite of the unfamiliar word. Thus, you are provided with some information that will bring you closer to defining the word. Consider the following example: *Despite his intelligence, Hector's low brow and bad posture made him look obtuse.* The author writes that Hector's appearance does not convey intelligence. Therefore, *obtuse* must mean unintelligent. Here is another example: *Despite the horrible weather, we were beatific about our trip to Alaska*. The word *despite* indicates that the speaker's feelings were at odds with the weather. Since the weather is described as *horrible*, then *beatific* must mean something positive.

Substitution to Find Meaning

In some cases, there will be very few contextual clues to help a reader define the meaning of an unfamiliar word. When this happens, one strategy that readers may employ is **substitution**. A good reader will brainstorm some possible synonyms for the given word, and he or she will substitute these words into the sentence. If the sentence and the surrounding passage continue to make sense, then the substitution has revealed at least some information about the unfamiliar word. Consider the sentence: *Frank's admonition rang in her ears as she climbed the mountain.* A reader unfamiliar with *admonition* might come up with some substitutions like *vow, promise, advice, complaint,* or *compliment.* All of these words make general sense of the sentence, though their meanings are diverse. However, this process has suggested that an admonition is some sort of message. The substitution strategy is rarely able to pinpoint a precise definition, but this process can be effective as a last resort.

Occasionally, you will be able to define an unfamiliar word by looking at the descriptive words in the context. Consider the following sentence: *Fred dragged the recalcitrant boy kicking and screaming up the stairs.* The words *dragged, kicking,* and *screaming* all suggest that the boy does not want to go up the stairs. The reader may assume that *recalcitrant* means something like unwilling or protesting. In this example, an unfamiliar adjective was identified.

Additionally, using description to define an unfamiliar noun is a common practice compared to unfamiliar adjectives, as in this sentence: *Don's wrinkled frown and constantly shaking fist identified him as a curmudgeon of the first order*. Don is described as having a *wrinkled frown and constantly shaking fist*, suggesting that a *curmudgeon* must be a grumpy person. Contrasts do not always provide detailed information about the unfamiliar word, but they at least give the reader some clues.

Words with Multiple Meanings

When a word has more than one meaning, readers can have difficulty determining how the word is being used in a given sentence. For instance, the verb *cleave*, can mean either *join* or *separate*. When readers come upon this word, they will have to select the definition that makes the most sense. Consider the following sentence: *Hermione's knife cleaved the bread cleanly*. Since a knife cannot join bread together, the word must indicate separation. A slightly more difficult example would be the sentence: *The birds cleaved to one another as they flew from the oak tree.* Immediately, the presence of the words *to one another* should suggest that in this sentence *cleave* is being used to mean *join*. Discovering the intent of a word with multiple meanings requires the same tricks as defining an unknown word: look for contextual clues and evaluate the substituted words.

Context Clues to Help Determine Meanings of Words

If readers simply bypass unknown words, they can reach unclear conclusions about what they read. However, looking for the definition of every unfamiliar word in the dictionary can slow their reading progress. Moreover, the dictionary may list multiple definitions for a word, so readers must search the word's context for meaning. Hence context is important to new vocabulary regardless of reader methods. Four types of context clues are examples, definitions, descriptive words, and opposites. Authors may use a certain word, and then follow it with several different examples of what it describes. Sometimes authors actually supply a definition of a word they use, which is especially true in informational and technical texts. Authors may use descriptive words that elaborate upon a vocabulary word they just used. Authors may also use opposites with negation that help define meaning.

Examples and Definitions

An author may use a word and then give examples that illustrate its meaning. Consider this text: "Teachers who do not know how to use sign language can help students who are deaf or hard of hearing understand certain instructions by using gestures instead, like pointing their fingers to indicate which direction to look or go; holding up a hand, palm outward, to indicate stopping; holding the hands flat, palms up, curling a finger toward oneself in a beckoning motion to indicate 'come here'; or curling all fingers toward oneself repeatedly to indicate 'come on', 'more', or 'continue.'" The author of this text has used the word "gestures" and then followed it with examples, so a reader unfamiliar with the word could deduce from the examples that "gestures" means "hand motions." Readers can find examples by looking for signal words "for example," "for instance," "like," "such as," and "e.g."

While readers sometimes have to look for definitions of unfamiliar words in a dictionary or do some work to determine a word's meaning from its surrounding context, at other times an author may make it easier for readers by defining certain words. For example, an author may write, "The company did not have sufficient capital, that is, available money, to continue operations." The author defined "capital" as "available money," and heralded the definition with the phrase "that is." Another way that authors supply word definitions is with appositives. Rather than being introduced by a signal phrase like "that is," "namely," or "meaning," an appositive comes after the vocabulary word it defines and is enclosed within two commas. For example, an author may write, "The Indians introduced the Pilgrims to pemmican, cakes they made of lean meat dried and mixed with fat, which proved greatly beneficial to keep settlers from starving while trapping." In this example, the appositive phrase following "pemmican" and preceding "which" defines the word "pemmican."

Descriptions

When readers encounter a word they do not recognize in a text, the author may expand on that word to illustrate it better. While the author may do this to make the prose more picturesque and vivid, the reader can also take advantage of this description to provide context clues to the meaning of the unfamiliar word. For example, an author may write, "The man sitting next to me on the airplane was obese. His shirt stretched across his vast expanse of flesh, strained almost to bursting." The descriptive second sentence elaborates on and helps to define the previous sentence's word "obese" to mean extremely fat. A reader unfamiliar with the word "repugnant" can decipher its meaning through an author's accompanying description: "The way the child grimaced and shuddered as he swallowed the medicine showed that its taste was particularly repugnant."

Opposites

Text authors sometimes introduce a contrasting or opposing idea before or after a concept they present. They may do this to emphasize or heighten the idea they present by contrasting it with something that is the reverse. However, readers can also use these context clues to understand familiar words. For example, an author may write, "Our conversation was not cheery. We sat and talked very solemnly about his experience and a number of similar events." The reader who is not familiar with the word "solemnly" can deduce by the author's preceding use of "not cheery" that "solemn" means the opposite of cheery or happy, so it must mean serious or sad. Or if someone writes, "Don't condemn his entire project because you couldn't find anything good to say about it," readers unfamiliar with "condemn" can understand from the sentence structure that it means the opposite of saying anything good, so it must mean reject, dismiss, or disapprove. "Entire" adds another context clue, meaning total or complete rejection.

Syntax to Determine Part of Speech and Meanings of Words

Syntax refers to sentence structure and word order. Suppose that a reader encounters an unfamiliar word when reading a text. To illustrate, consider an invented word like "splunch." If this word is used in a sentence like "Please splunch that ball to me," the reader can assume from syntactic context that "splunch" is a verb. We would not use a noun, adjective, adverb, or preposition with the object "that ball," and the prepositional phrase "to me" further indicates "splunch" represents an action. However, in the sentence, "Please hand that splunch to me," the reader can assume that "splunch" is a noun. Demonstrative adjectives like "that" modify nouns. Also, we hand someone some*thing*—a thing being a noun; we do not hand someone a verb, adjective, or adverb. Some sentences contain further clues. For example, from the sentence, "The princess wore the glittering splunch on her head," the reader can deduce that it is a crown, tiara, or something similar from the syntactic context, without knowing the word.

Syntax to Indicate Different Meanings of Similar Sentences

The syntax, or structure, of a sentence affords grammatical cues that aid readers in comprehending the meanings of words, phrases, and sentences in the texts that they read. Seemingly minor differences in how the words or phrases in a sentence are ordered can make major differences in meaning. For example, two sentences can use exactly the same words but have different meanings based on the word order:

- "The man with a broken arm sat in a chair."
- "The man sat in a chair with a broken arm."

While both sentences indicate that a man sat in a chair, differing syntax indicates whether the man's or chair's arm was broken.

Review Video: Syntax
Visit mometrix.com/academy and enter code: 242280

Determining Meaning of Phrases and Paragraphs

Like unknown words, the meanings of phrases, paragraphs, and entire works can also be difficult to discern. Each of these can be better understood with added context. However, for larger groups of words, more context is needed. Unclear phrases are similar to unclear words, and the same methods can be used to understand their meaning. However, it is also important to consider how the individual words in the phrase work together. Paragraphs are a bit more complicated. Just as words must be compared to other words in a sentence, paragraphs must be compared to other paragraphs in a composition or a section.

Determining Meaning in Various Types of Compositions

To understand the meaning of an entire composition, the type of composition must be considered. **Expository writing** is generally organized so that each paragraph focuses on explaining one idea, or part of an idea, and its relevance. **Persuasive writing** uses paragraphs for different purposes to organize the parts of the argument. **Unclear paragraphs** must be read in the context of the paragraphs around them for their meaning to be fully understood. The meaning of full texts can also be unclear at times. The purpose of composition is also important for understanding the meaning of a text. To quickly understand the broad meaning of a text, look to the introductory and concluding paragraphs. Fictional texts are different. Some fictional works have implicit meanings, but some do not. The target audience must be considered for understanding texts that do have an implicit meaning, as most children's fiction will clearly state any lessons or morals. For other fiction, the application of literary theories and criticism may be helpful for understanding the text.

Resources for Determining Word Meaning and Usage

While these strategies are useful for determining the meaning of unknown words and phrases, sometimes additional resources are needed to properly use the terms in different contexts. Some words have multiple definitions, and some words are inappropriate in particular contexts or modes of writing. The following tools are helpful for understanding all meanings and proper uses for words and phrases.

- **Dictionaries** provide the meaning of a multitude of words in a language. Many dictionaries include additional information about each word, such as its etymology, its synonyms, or variations of the word.
- **Glossaries** are similar to dictionaries, as they provide the meanings of a variety of terms. However, while dictionaries typically feature an extensive list of words and comprise an entire publication, glossaries are often included at the end of a text and only include terms and definitions that are relevant to the text they follow.
- **Spell Checkers** are used to detect spelling errors in typed text. Some spell checkers may also detect the misuse of plural or singular nouns, verb tenses, or capitalization. While spell checkers are a helpful tool, they are not always reliable or attuned to the author's intent, so it is important to review the spell checker's suggestions before accepting them.
- **Style Manuals** are guidelines on the preferred punctuation, format, and grammar usage according to different fields or organizations. For example, the Associated Press Stylebook is a style guide often used for media writing. The guidelines within a style guide are not

always applicable across different contexts and usages, as the guidelines often cover grammatical or formatting situations that are not objectively correct or incorrect.

Main Ideas and Supporting Details

Identifying Topics and Main Ideas

One of the most important skills in reading comprehension is the identification of **topics** and **main ideas**. There is a subtle difference between these two features. The topic is the subject of a text (i.e., what the text is all about). The main idea, on the other hand, is the most important point being made by the author. The topic is usually expressed in a few words at the most while the main idea often needs a full sentence to be completely defined. As an example, a short passage might be written on the topic of penguins, and the main idea could be written as *Penguins are different from other birds in many ways*. In most nonfiction writing, the topic and the main idea will be **stated directly** and often appear in a sentence at the very beginning or end of the text. When being tested on an understanding of the author's topic, you may be able to skim the passage for the general idea by reading only the first sentence of each paragraph. A body paragraph's first sentence is often—but not always—the main **topic sentence** which gives you a summary of the content in the paragraph.

However, there are cases in which the reader must figure out an **unstated** topic or main idea. In these instances, you must read every sentence of the text and try to come up with an overarching idea that is supported by each of those sentences.

Note: The main idea should not be confused with the thesis statement. While the main idea gives a brief, general summary of a text, the thesis statement provides a **specific perspective** on an issue that the author supports with evidence.

Review Video: Topics and Main Ideas
Visit mometrix.com/academy and enter code: 407801

Supporting Details

Supporting details are smaller pieces of evidence that provide backing for the main point. In order to show that a main idea is correct or valid, an author must add details that prove their point. All texts contain details, but they are only classified as supporting details when they serve to reinforce some larger point. Supporting details are most commonly found in informative and persuasive texts. In some cases, they will be clearly indicated with terms like *for example* or *for instance*, or they will be enumerated with terms like *first*, *second*, and *last*. However, you need to be prepared for texts that do not contain those indicators. As a reader, you should consider whether the author's supporting details really back up his or her main point. Details can be factual and correct, yet they may not be **relevant** to the author's point. Conversely, details can be relevant, but be ineffective because they are based on opinion or assertions that cannot be proven.

Review Video: Supporting Details
Visit mometrix.com/academy and enter code: 396297

Author's Purpose

Author's Purpose

Usually, identifying the author's **purpose** is easier than identifying his or her **position**. In most cases, the author has no interest in hiding his or her purpose. A text that is meant to entertain, for instance, should be written to please the reader. Most narratives, or stories, are written to entertain, though they may also inform or persuade. Informative texts are easy to identify, while the most difficult purpose of a text to identify is persuasion because the author has an interest in making this purpose hard to detect. When a reader discovers that the author is trying to persuade, he or she should be skeptical of the argument. For this reason, persuasive texts often try to establish an entertaining tone and hope to amuse the reader into agreement. On the other hand, an informative tone may be implemented to create an appearance of authority and objectivity.

An author's purpose is evident often in the **organization** of the text (e.g., section headings in bold font points to an informative text). However, you may not have such organization available to you in your exam. Instead, if the author makes his or her main idea clear from the beginning, then the likely purpose of the text is to **inform**. If the author begins by making a claim and provides various arguments to support that claim, then the purpose is probably to **persuade**. If the author tells a story or wants to gain the reader's attention more than to push a particular point or deliver information, then his or her purpose is most likely to **entertain**. As a reader, you must judge authors on how well they accomplish their purpose. In other words, you need to consider the type of passage (e.g., technical, persuasive, etc.) that the author has written and if the author has followed the requirements of the passage type.

Review Video: Understanding the Author's Intent
Visit mometrix.com/academy and enter code: 511819

Informational Texts

An **informational text** is written to educate and enlighten readers. Informational texts are almost always nonfiction and are rarely structured as a story. The intention of an informational text is to deliver information in the most comprehensible way. So, look for the structure of the text to be very clear. In an informational text, the thesis statement is one or two sentences that normally appears at the end of the first paragraph. The author may use some colorful language, but he or she is likely to put more emphasis on clarity and precision. Informational essays do not typically appeal to the emotions. They often contain facts and figures and rarely include the opinion of the author; however, readers should remain aware of the possibility for bias as those facts are presented. Sometimes a persuasive essay can resemble an informative essay, especially if the author maintains an even tone and presents his or her views as if they were established fact.

Review Video: Informational Text
Visit mometrix.com/academy and enter code: 924964

Persuasive Writing

In a persuasive essay, the author is attempting to change the reader's mind or **convince** him or her of something that he or she did not believe previously. There are several identifying characteristics of **persuasive writing**. One is **opinion presented as fact**. When authors attempt to persuade readers, they often present their opinions as if they were fact. Readers must be on guard for statements that sound factual but which cannot be subjected to research, observation, or experiment. Another characteristic of persuasive writing is **emotional language**. An author will often try to play on the emotions of readers by appealing to their sympathy or sense of morality.

When an author uses colorful or evocative language with the intent of arousing the reader's passions, then the author may be attempting to persuade. Finally, in many cases, a persuasive text will give an **unfair explanation of opposing positions**, if these positions are mentioned at all.

Entertaining Texts

The success or failure of an author's intent to **entertain** is determined by those who read the author's work. Entertaining texts may be either fiction or nonfiction, and they may describe real or imagined people, places, and events. Entertaining texts are often narratives or poems. A text that is written to entertain is likely to contain **colorful language** that engages the imagination and the emotions. Such writing often features a great deal of figurative language, which typically enlivens the subject matter with images and analogies.

Though an entertaining text is not usually written to persuade or inform, authors may accomplish both of these tasks in their work. An entertaining text may *appeal to the reader's emotions* and cause him or her to think differently about a particular subject. In any case, entertaining texts tend to showcase the personality of the author more than other types of writing.

Descriptive Text

In a sense, almost all writing is descriptive, insofar as an author seeks to describe events, ideas, or people to the reader. Some texts, however, are primarily concerned with **description**. A descriptive text focuses on a particular subject and attempts to depict the subject in a way that will be clear to readers. Descriptive texts contain many adjectives and adverbs (i.e., words that give shades of meaning and create a more detailed mental picture for the reader). A descriptive text fails when it is unclear to the reader. A descriptive text will certainly be informative and may be persuasive and entertaining as well.

Review Video: Descriptive Texts
Visit mometrix.com/academy and enter code: 174903

Expression of Feelings

When an author intends to **express feelings**, he or she may use **expressive and bold language**. An author may write with emotion for any number of reasons. Sometimes, authors will express feelings because they are describing a personal situation of great pain or happiness. In other situations, authors will attempt to persuade the reader and will use emotion to stir up the passions. This kind of expression is easy to identify when the writer uses phrases like *I felt* and *I sense*. However, readers may find that the author will simply describe feelings without introducing them. As a reader, you must know the importance of recognizing when an author is expressing emotion and not to become overwhelmed by sympathy or passion. Readers should maintain some **detachment** so that they can still evaluate the strength of the author's argument or the quality of the writing.

Review Video: Emotional Language in Literature
Visit mometrix.com/academy and enter code: 759390

Expository Passage

An **expository** passage aims to **inform** and enlighten readers. Expository passages are nonfiction and usually center around a simple, easily defined topic. Since the goal of exposition is to teach, such a passage should be as clear as possible. Often, an expository passage contains helpful organizing words, like *first*, *next*, *for example*, and *therefore*. These words keep the reader **oriented** in the text. Although expository passages do not need to feature colorful language and artful writing, they are often more effective with these features. For a reader, the challenge of expository passages is to maintain steady attention. Expository passages are not always about subjects that will naturally interest a reader, so the writer is often more concerned with **clarity** and **comprehensibility** than with engaging the reader. By reading actively, you can ensure a good habit of focus when reading an expository passage.

Review Video: Expository Passages
Visit mometrix.com/academy and enter code: 256515

Narrative Passage

A **narrative** passage is a story that can be fiction or nonfiction. However, there are a few elements that a text must have in order to be classified as a narrative. First, the text must have a **plot** (i.e., a series of events). Narratives often proceed in a clear sequence, but this is not a requirement. If the narrative is good, then these events will be interesting to readers. Second, a narrative has **characters**. These characters could be people, animals, or even inanimate objects—so long as they participate in the plot. Third, a narrative passage often contains **figurative language** which is meant to stimulate the imagination of readers by making comparisons and observations. For instance, a *metaphor*, a common piece of figurative language, is a description of one thing in terms of another. *The moon was a frosty snowball* is an example of a metaphor. In the literal sense this is obviously untrue, but the comparison suggests a certain mood for the reader.

Technical Passage

A **technical** passage is written to *describe* a complex object or process. Technical writing is common in medical and technological fields, in which complex ideas of mathematics, science, and engineering need to be explained *simply* and *clearly*. To ease comprehension, a technical passage usually proceeds in a very logical order. Technical passages often have clear headings and subheadings, which are used to keep the reader oriented in the text. Additionally, you will find that these passages divide sections up with numbers or letters. Many technical passages look more like an outline than a piece of prose. The amount of **jargon** or difficult vocabulary will vary in a technical passage depending on the intended audience. As much as possible, technical passages try to avoid language that the reader will have to research in order to understand the message, yet readers will find that jargon cannot always be avoided.

Review Video: Technical Passages
Visit mometrix.com/academy and enter code: 478923

Common Organizations of Texts

Organization of the Text

The way a text is organized can help readers understand the author's intent and his or her conclusions. There are various ways to organize a text, and each one has a purpose and use. Usually, authors will organize information logically in a passage so the reader can follow and locate the information within the text. However, since not all passages are written with the same logical structure, you need to be familiar with several different types of passage structure.

Review Video: Sequence of Events in a Story
Visit mometrix.com/academy and enter code: 807512

CHRONOLOGICAL

When using **chronological** order, the author presents information in the order that it happened. For example, biographies are typically written in chronological order. The subject's birth and childhood are presented first, followed by their adult life, and lastly the events leading up to the person's death.

CAUSE AND EFFECT

One of the most common text structures is **cause and effect**. A **cause** is an act or event that makes something happen, and an **effect** is the thing that happens as a result of the cause. A cause-and-effect relationship is not always explicit, but there are some terms in English that signal causes, such as *since*, *because*, and *due to*. Furthermore, terms that signal effects include *consequently, therefore, this leads to*. As an example, consider the sentence *Because the sky was clear, Ron did not bring an umbrella*. The cause is the clear sky, and the effect is that Ron did not bring an umbrella. However, readers may find that sometimes the cause-and-effect relationship will not be clearly noted. For instance, the sentence *He was late and missed the meeting* does not contain any signaling words, but the sentence still contains a cause (he was late) and an effect (he missed the meeting).

Review Video: Cause and Effect
Visit mometrix.com/academy and enter code: 868099

Review Video: Rhetorical Strategy of Cause and Effect Analysis
Visit mometrix.com/academy and enter code: 725944

MULTIPLE EFFECTS

Be aware of the possibility for a single cause to have **multiple effects.** (e.g., *Single cause*: Because you left your homework on the table, your dog engulfed the assignment. *Multiple effects*: As a result, you receive a failing grade, your parents do not allow you to go out with your friends, you miss out on the new movie, and one of your classmates spoils it for you before you have another chance to watch it).

MULTIPLE CAUSES

Also, there is the possibility for a single effect to have **multiple causes.** (e.g., *Single effect*: Alan has a fever. *Multiple causes*: An unexpected cold front came through the area, and Alan forgot to take his multi-vitamin to avoid getting sick.) Additionally, an effect can in turn be the cause of another effect, in what is known as a cause-and-effect chain. (e.g., As a result of her disdain for procrastination, Lynn prepared for her exam. This led to her passing her test with high marks. Hence, her resume was accepted and her application was approved.)

CAUSE AND EFFECT IN PERSUASIVE ESSAYS

Persuasive essays, in which an author tries to make a convincing argument and change the minds of readers, usually include cause-and-effect relationships. However, these relationships should not always be taken at face value. Frequently, an author will assume a cause or take an effect for granted. To read a persuasive essay effectively, readers need to judge the cause-and-effect relationships that the author is presenting. For instance, imagine an author wrote the following: *The parking deck has been unprofitable because people would prefer to ride their bikes.* The relationship is clear: the cause is that people prefer to ride their bikes, and the effect is that the parking deck has been unprofitable. However, readers should consider whether this argument is conclusive. Perhaps there are other reasons for the failure of the parking deck: a down economy, excessive fees, etc. Too often, authors present causal relationships as if they are fact rather than opinion. Readers should be on the alert for these dubious claims.

Problem-Solution

Some nonfiction texts are organized to **present a problem** followed by a solution. For this type of text, the problem is often explained before the solution is offered. In some cases, as when the problem is well known, the solution may be introduced briefly at the beginning. Other passages may focus on the solution, and the problem will be referenced only occasionally. Some texts will outline multiple solutions to a problem, leaving readers to choose among them. If the author has an interest or an allegiance to one solution, he or she may fail to mention or describe accurately some of the other solutions. Readers should be careful of the author's agenda when reading a problem-solution text. Only by understanding the author's perspective and interests can one develop a proper judgment of the proposed solution.

Compare and Contrast

Many texts follow the **compare-and-contrast** model in which the similarities and differences between two ideas or things are explored. Analysis of the similarities between ideas is called **comparison**. In an ideal comparison, the author places ideas or things in an equivalent structure, i.e., the author presents the ideas in the same way. If an author wants to show the similarities between cricket and baseball, then he or she may do so by summarizing the equipment and rules for each game. Be mindful of the similarities as they appear in the passage and take note of any differences that are mentioned. Often, these small differences will only reinforce the more general similarity.

Review Video: Compare and Contrast
Visit mometrix.com/academy and enter code: 798319

Thinking critically about ideas and conclusions can seem like a daunting task. One way to ease this task is to understand the basic elements of ideas and writing techniques. Looking at the ways different ideas relate to each other can be a good way for readers to begin their analysis. For instance, sometimes authors will write about two ideas that are in opposition to each other. Or, one author will provide his or her ideas on a topic, and another author may respond in opposition. The analysis of these opposing ideas is known as **contrast**. Contrast is often marred by the author's obvious partiality to one of the ideas. A discerning reader will be put off by an author who does not engage in a fair fight. In an analysis of opposing ideas, both ideas should be presented in clear and reasonable terms. If the author does prefer a side, you need to read carefully to determine the areas where the author shows or avoids this preference. In an analysis of opposing ideas, you should proceed through the passage by marking the major differences point by point with an eye that is looking for an explanation of each side's view. For instance, in an analysis of capitalism and communism, there is an importance in outlining each side's view on labor, markets, prices, personal responsibility, etc. Additionally, as you read through the passages, you should note whether the opposing views present each side in a similar manner.

Sequence

Readers must be able to identify a text's **sequence**, or the order in which things happen. Often, when the sequence is very important to the author, the text is indicated with signal words like *first, then, next,* and *last*. However, a sequence can be merely implied and must be noted by the reader. Consider the sentence *He walked through the garden and gave water and fertilizer to the plants.* Clearly, the man did not walk through the garden before he collected water and fertilizer for the plants. So, the implied sequence is that he first collected water, then he collected fertilizer, next he walked through the garden, and last he gave water or fertilizer as necessary to the plants. Texts do not always proceed in an orderly sequence from first to last. Sometimes they begin at the end and start over at the beginning. As a reader, you can enhance your understanding of the passage by taking brief notes to clarify the sequence.

Review Video: Sequence
Visit mometrix.com/academy and enter code: 489027

Making and Evaluating Predictions

Making Predictions

When we read literature, **making predictions** about what will happen in the writing reinforces our purpose for reading and prepares us mentally. A **prediction** is a guess about what will happen next. Readers constantly make predictions based on what they have read and what they already know. We can make predictions before we begin reading and during our reading. Consider the following sentence: *Staring at the computer screen in shock, Kim blindly reached over for the brimming glass of water on the shelf to her side.* The sentence suggests that Kim is distracted, and that she is not looking at the glass that she is going to pick up. So, a reader might predict that Kim is going to knock over the glass. Of course, not every prediction will be accurate: perhaps Kim will pick the glass up cleanly. Nevertheless, the author has certainly created the expectation that the water might be spilled.

As we read on, we can test the accuracy of our predictions, revise them in light of additional reading, and confirm or refute our predictions. Predictions are always subject to revision as the reader acquires more information. A reader can make predictions by observing the title and illustrations; noting the structure, characters, and subject; drawing on existing knowledge relative to the subject; and asking "why" and "who" questions. Connecting reading to what we already know enables us to learn new information and construct meaning. For example, before third-graders read a book about Johnny Appleseed, they may start a KWL chart—a list of what they *Know*, what they *Want* to know or learn, and what they have *Learned* after reading. Activating existing background knowledge and thinking about the text before reading improves comprehension.

Review Video: Predictive Reading
Visit mometrix.com/academy and enter code: 437248

Test-taking tip: To respond to questions requiring future predictions, your answers should be based on evidence of past or present behavior and events.

Evaluating Predictions

When making predictions, readers should be able to explain how they developed their prediction. One way readers can defend their thought process is by citing textual evidence. Textual evidence to evaluate reader predictions about literature includes specific synopses of the work, paraphrases of the work or parts of it, and direct quotations from the work. These references to the text must support the prediction by indicating, clearly or unclearly, what will happen later in the story. A text may provide these indications through literary devices such as foreshadowing. Foreshadowing is anything in a text that gives the reader a hint about what is to come by emphasizing the likelihood of an event or development. Foreshadowing can occur through descriptions, exposition, and dialogue. Foreshadowing in dialogue usually occurs when a character gives a warning or expresses a strong feeling that a certain event will occur. Foreshadowing can also occur through irony. However, unlike other forms of foreshadowing, the events that seem the most likely are the opposite of what actually happens. Instances of foreshadowing and irony can be summarized, paraphrased, or quoted to defend a reader's prediction.

Review Video: Textual Evidence for Predictions
Visit mometrix.com/academy and enter code: 261070

Making Inferences and Drawing Conclusions

Inferences are logical conclusions that readers make based on their observations and previous knowledge. An inference is based on both what is found in a passage or a story and what is known from personal experience. For instance, a story may say that a character is frightened and can hear howling in the distance. Based on both what is in the text and personal knowledge, it is a logical conclusion that the character is frightened because he hears the sound of wolves. A good inference is supported by the information in a passage.

Implicit and Explicit Information

By inferring, readers construct meanings from text that are personally relevant. By combining their own schemas or concepts and their background information pertinent to the text with what they read, readers interpret it according to both what the author has conveyed and their own unique perspectives. Inferences are different from **explicit information**, which is clearly stated in a passage. Authors do not always explicitly spell out every meaning in what they write; many meanings are implicit. Through inference, readers can comprehend implied meanings in the text, and also derive personal significance from it, making the text meaningful and memorable to them. Inference is a natural process in everyday life. When readers infer, they can draw conclusions about what the author is saying, predict what may reasonably follow, amend these predictions as they continue to read, interpret the import of themes, and analyze the characters' feelings and motivations through their actions.

Example of Drawing Conclusions from Inferences

Read the excerpt and decide why Jana finally relaxed.

> Jana loved her job, but the work was very demanding. She had trouble relaxing. She called a friend, but she still thought about work. She ordered a pizza, but eating it did not help. Then, her kitten jumped on her lap and began to purr. Jana leaned back and began to hum a little tune. She felt better.

You can draw the conclusion that Jana relaxed because her kitten jumped on her lap. The kitten purred, and Jana leaned back and hummed a tune. Then she felt better. The excerpt does not explicitly say that this is the reason why she was able to relax. The text leaves the matter unclear, but the reader can infer or make a "best guess" that this is the reason she is relaxing. This is a logical conclusion based on the information in the passage. It is the best conclusion a reader can make based on the information he or she has read. Inferences are based on the information in a passage, but they are not directly stated in the passage.

Test-taking tip: While being tested on your ability to make correct inferences, you must look for **contextual clues**. An answer can be true, but not the best or most correct answer. The contextual clues will help you find the answer that is the **best answer** out of the given choices. Be careful in your reading to understand the context in which a phrase is stated. When asked for the implied meaning of a statement made in the passage, you should immediately locate the statement and read the **context** in which the statement was made. Also, look for an answer choice that has a similar phrase to the statement in question.

Review Video: Inference
Visit mometrix.com/academy and enter code: 379203

Review Video: How to Support a Conclusion
Visit mometrix.com/academy and enter code: 281653

Critical Reading Skills

Opinions, Facts, and Fallacies

Critical thinking skills are mastered through understanding various types of writing and the different purposes authors can have for writing different passages. Every author writes for a purpose. When you understand their purpose and how they accomplish their goal, you will be able to analyze their writing and determine whether or not you agree with their conclusions.

Readers must always be aware of the difference between fact and opinion. A **fact** can be subjected to analysis and proven to be true. An **opinion**, on the other hand, is the author's personal thoughts or feelings and may not be altered by research or evidence. If the author writes that the distance from New York City to Boston is about two hundred miles, then he or she is stating a fact. If the author writes that New York City is too crowded, then he or she is giving an opinion because there is no objective standard for overpopulation. Opinions are often supported by facts. For instance, an author might use a comparison between the population density of New York City and that of other major American cities as evidence of an overcrowded population. An opinion supported by facts tends to be more convincing. On the other hand, when authors support their opinions with other opinions, readers should employ critical thinking and approach the argument with skepticism.

Review Video: Distinguishing Fact and Opinion
Visit mometrix.com/academy and enter code: 870899

Reliable Sources

When you read an argumentative passage, you need to be sure that facts are presented to the reader from **reliable sources**. An opinion is what the author thinks about a given topic. An opinion is not common knowledge or proven by expert sources, instead the information is the personal beliefs and thoughts of the author. To distinguish between fact and opinion, a reader needs to consider the type of source that is presenting information, the information that backs-up a claim, and the author's motivation to have a certain point-of-view on a given topic. For example, if a panel of scientists has conducted multiple studies on the effectiveness of taking a certain vitamin, then the results are more likely to be factual than those of a company that is selling a vitamin and simply claims that taking the vitamin can produce positive effects. The company is motivated to sell their product, and the scientists are using the scientific method to prove a theory. Remember, if you find sentences that contain phrases such as "I think...", then the statement is an opinion.

Biases

In their attempts to persuade, writers often make mistakes in their thought processes and writing choices. These processes and choices are important to understand so you can make an informed decision about the author's credibility. Every author has a point of view, but authors demonstrate a **bias** when they ignore reasonable counterarguments or distort opposing viewpoints. A bias is evident whenever the author's claims are presented in a way that is unfair or inaccurate. Bias can be intentional or unintentional, but readers should be skeptical of the author's argument in either case. Remember that a biased author may still be correct. However, the author will be correct in spite of, not because of, his or her bias.

A **stereotype** is a bias applied specifically to a group of people or a place. Stereotyping is considered to be particularly abhorrent because it promotes negative, misleading generalizations about people. Readers should be very cautious of authors who use stereotypes in their writing. These faulty assumptions typically reveal the author's ignorance and lack of curiosity.

Review Video: Bias and Stereotype
Visit mometrix.com/academy and enter code: 644829

Persuasion and Rhetoric

Persuasive Techniques

To **appeal using reason**, writers present logical arguments, such as using "If... then... because" statements. To **appeal to emotions**, authors may ask readers how they would feel about something or to put themselves in another's place, present their argument as one that will make the audience feel good, or tell readers how they should feel. To **appeal to character**, **morality**, or **ethics**, authors present their points to readers as the right or most moral choices. Authors cite expert opinions to show readers that someone very knowledgeable about the subject or viewpoint agrees with the author's claims. **Testimonials**, usually via anecdotes or quotations regarding the author's subject, help build the audience's trust in an author's message through positive support from ordinary people. **Bandwagon appeals** claim that everybody else agrees with the author's argument and persuade readers to conform and agree, also. Authors **appeal to greed** by presenting their choice as cheaper, free, or more valuable for less cost. They **appeal to laziness** by presenting their views as more convenient, easy, or relaxing. Authors also anticipate potential objections and argue against them before audiences think of them, thereby depicting those objections as weak.

Authors can use **comparisons** like analogies, similes, and metaphors to persuade audiences. For example, a writer might represent excessive expenses as "hemorrhaging" money, which the author's recommended solution will stop. Authors can use negative word connotations to make some choices unappealing to readers, and positive word connotations to make others more appealing. Using **humor** can relax readers and garner their agreement. However, writers must take care: ridiculing opponents can be a successful strategy for appealing to readers who already agree with the author, but can backfire by angering other readers. **Rhetorical questions** need no answer, but create effect that can force agreement, such as asking the question, "Wouldn't you rather be paid more than less?" **Generalizations** persuade readers by being impossible to disagree with. Writers can easily make generalizations that appear to support their viewpoints, like saying, "We all want peace, not war" regarding more specific political arguments. **Transfer** and **association** persuade by example: if advertisements show attractive actors enjoying their products, audiences imagine they will experience the same. **Repetition** can also sometimes effectively persuade audiences.

Review Video: Using Rhetorical Strategies for Persuasion
Visit mometrix.com/academy and enter code: 302658

Classical Author Appeals

In his *On Rhetoric,* ancient Greek philosopher Aristotle defined three basic types of appeal used in writing, which he called *pathos*, *ethos*, and *logos*. ***Pathos*** means suffering or experience and refers to appeals to the emotions (the English word *pathetic* comes from this root). Writing that is meant to entertain audiences, by making them either happy, as with comedy, or sad, as with tragedy, uses *pathos*. Aristotle's *Poetics* states that evoking the emotions of terror and pity is one of the criteria for writing tragedy. ***Ethos*** means character and connotes ideology (the English word *ethics* comes from this root). Writing that appeals to credibility, based on academic, professional, or personal merit, uses *ethos*. ***Logos*** means "I say" and refers to a plea, opinion, expectation, word or speech, account, opinion, or reason (the English word *logic* comes from this root.) Aristotle used it to mean persuasion that appeals to the audience through reasoning and logic to influence their opinions.

Rhetorical Devices

- An **anecdote** is a brief story authors may relate to their argument, which can illustrate their points in a more real and relatable way.
- **Aphorisms** concisely state common beliefs and may rhyme. For example, Benjamin Franklin's "Early to bed and early to rise / Makes a man healthy, wealthy, and wise" is an aphorism.
- **Allusions** refer to literary or historical figures to impart symbolism to a thing or person and to create reader resonance. In John Steinbeck's *Of Mice and Men*, protagonist George's last name is Milton. This alludes to John Milton, who wrote *Paradise Lost*, and symbolizes George's eventual loss of his dream.
- **Satire** exaggerates, ridicules, or pokes fun at human flaws or ideas, as in the works of Jonathan Swift and Mark Twain.
- A **parody** is a form of satire that imitates another work to ridicule its topic or style.
- A **paradox** is a statement that is true despite appearing contradictory.
- **Hyperbole** is overstatement using exaggerated language.
- An **oxymoron** combines seeming contradictions, such as "deafening silence."
- **Analogies** compare two things that share common elements.
- **Similes** (stated comparisons using the words *like* or *as*) and **metaphors** (stated comparisons that do not use *like* or *as*) are considered forms of analogy.
- When using logic to reason with audiences, **syllogism** refers either to deductive reasoning or a deceptive, very sophisticated, or subtle argument.
- **Deductive reasoning** moves from general to specific, **inductive reasoning** from specific to general.
- **Diction** is author word choice that establishes tone and effect.
- **Understatement** achieves effects like contrast or irony by downplaying or describing something more subtly than warranted.
- **Chiasmus** uses parallel clauses, the second reversing the order of the first. Examples include T. S. Eliot's "Has the Church failed mankind, or has mankind failed the Church?" and John F. Kennedy's "Ask not what your country can do for you; ask what you can do for your country."
- **Anaphora** regularly repeats a word or phrase at the beginnings of consecutive clauses or phrases to add emphasis to an idea. A classic example of anaphora was Winston Churchill's emphasis of determination: "[W]e shall fight on the beaches, we shall fight on the landing grounds, we shall fight in the fields and in the streets, we shall fight in the hills; we shall never surrender..."

Reading Informational Texts

Language Use

Literal and Figurative Language

As in fictional literature, informational text also uses both **literal language**, which means just what it says, and **figurative language**, which imparts more than literal meaning. For example, an informational text author might use a simile or direct comparison, such as writing that a racehorse "ran like the wind." Informational text authors also use metaphors or implied comparisons, such as "the cloud of the Great Depression." Imagery may also appear in informational texts to increase the reader's understanding of ideas and concepts discussed in the text.

Review Video: Figurative Language
Visit mometrix.com/academy and enter code: 584902

Explicit and Implicit Information

When informational text states something explicitly, the reader is told by the author exactly what is meant, which can include the author's interpretation or perspective of events. For example, a professor writes, "I have seen students go into an absolute panic just because they weren't able to complete the exam in the time they were allotted." This explicitly tells the reader that the students were afraid, and by using the words "just because," the writer indicates their fear was exaggerated out of proportion relative to what happened. However, another professor writes, "I have had students come to me, their faces drained of all color, saying 'We weren't able to finish the exam.'" This is an example of implicit meaning: the second writer did not state explicitly that the students were panicked. Instead, he wrote a description of their faces being "drained of all color." From this description, the reader can infer that the students were so frightened that their faces paled.

Review Video: Explicit and Implicit Information
Visit mometrix.com/academy and enter code: 735771

Making Inferences About Informational Text

With informational text, reader comprehension depends not only on recalling important statements and details, but also on reader inferences based on examples and details. Readers add information from the text to what they already know to draw inferences about the text. These inferences help the readers to fill in the information that the text does not explicitly state, enabling them to understand the text better. When reading a nonfictional autobiography or biography, for example, the most appropriate inferences might concern the events in the book, the actions of the subject of the autobiography or biography, and the message the author means to convey. When reading a nonfictional expository (informational) text, the reader would best draw inferences about problems and their solutions, and causes and their effects. When reading a nonfictional persuasive text, the reader will want to infer ideas supporting the author's message and intent.

Structures or Organizational Patterns in Informational Texts

Informational text can be **descriptive**, appealing to the five senses and answering the questions what, who, when, where, and why. Another method of structuring informational text is sequence and order. **Chronological** texts relate events in the sequence that they occurred, from start to finish, while how-to texts organize information into a series of instructions in the sequence in which the steps should be followed. **Comparison-contrast** structures of informational text describe various ideas to their readers by pointing out how things or ideas are similar and how they are different. **Cause and effect** structures of informational text describe events that occurred and identify the causes or reasons that those events occurred. **Problem and solution** structures of informational texts introduce and describe problems and offer one or more solutions for each problem described.

DETERMINING AN INFORMATIONAL AUTHOR'S PURPOSE

Informational authors' purposes are why they write texts. Readers must determine authors' motivations and goals. Readers gain greater insight into a text by considering the author's motivation. This develops critical reading skills. Readers perceive writing as a person's voice, not simply printed words. Uncovering author motivations and purposes empowers readers to know what to expect from the text, read for relevant details, evaluate authors and their work critically, and respond effectively to the motivations and persuasions of the text. The main idea of a text is what the reader is supposed to understand from reading it; the purpose of the text is why the author has written it and what the author wants readers to do with its information. Authors state some purposes clearly, while other purposes may be unstated but equally significant. When stated purposes contradict other parts of a text, the author may have a hidden agenda. Readers can better evaluate a text's effectiveness, whether they agree or disagree with it, and why they agree or disagree through identifying unstated author purposes.

IDENTIFYING AUTHOR'S POINT OF VIEW OR PURPOSE

In some informational texts, readers find it easy to identify the author's point of view and purpose, such as when the author explicitly states his or her position and reason for writing. But other texts are more difficult, either because of the content or because the authors give neutral or balanced viewpoints. This is particularly true in scientific texts, in which authors may state the purpose of their research in the report, but never state their point of view except by interpreting evidence or data.

To analyze text and identify point of view or purpose, readers should ask themselves the following four questions:

1. With what main point or idea does this author want to persuade readers to agree?
2. How does this author's word choice affect the way that readers consider this subject?
3. How do this author's choices of examples and facts affect the way that readers consider this subject?
4. What is it that this author wants to accomplish by writing this text?

Review Video: Understanding the Author's Intent
Visit mometrix.com/academy and enter code: 511819

Review Video: Author's Position
Visit mometrix.com/academy and enter code: 827954

EVALUATING ARGUMENTS MADE BY INFORMATIONAL TEXT WRITERS

When evaluating an informational text, the first step is to identify the argument's conclusion. Then identify the author's premises that support the conclusion. Try to paraphrase premises for clarification and make the conclusion and premises fit. List all premises first, sequentially numbered, then finish with the conclusion. Identify any premises or assumptions not stated by the author but required for the stated premises to support the conclusion. Read word assumptions sympathetically, as the author might. Evaluate whether premises reasonably support the conclusion. For inductive reasoning, the reader should ask if the premises are true, if they support the conclusion, and if so, how strongly. For deductive reasoning, the reader should ask if the argument is valid or invalid. If all premises are true, then the argument is valid unless the conclusion can be false. If it can, then the argument is invalid. An invalid argument can be made valid through alterations such as the addition of needed premises.

USE OF RHETORIC IN INFORMATIONAL TEXTS

There are many ways authors can support their claims, arguments, beliefs, ideas, and reasons for writing in informational texts. For example, authors can appeal to readers' sense of **logic** by communicating their reasoning through a carefully sequenced series of logical steps to help "prove" the points made. Authors can appeal to readers' **emotions** by using descriptions and words that evoke feelings of sympathy, sadness, anger, righteous indignation, hope, happiness, or any other emotion to reinforce what they express and share with their audience. Authors may appeal to the **moral** or **ethical values** of readers by using words and descriptions that can convince readers that something is right or wrong. By relating personal anecdotes, authors can supply readers with more accessible, realistic examples of points they make, as well as appealing to their emotions. They can provide supporting evidence by reporting case studies. They can also illustrate their points by making analogies to which readers can better relate.

Organizational Features in Texts

TEXT FEATURES IN INFORMATIONAL TEXTS

- The **title of a text** gives readers some idea of its content.
- The **table of contents** is a list near the beginning of a text, showing the book's sections and chapters and their coinciding page numbers. This gives readers an overview of the whole text and helps them find specific chapters easily.
- An **appendix**, at the back of the book or document, includes important information that is not present in the main text.
- Also at the back, an **index** lists the book's important topics alphabetically with their page numbers to help readers find them easily.
- **Glossaries**, usually found at the backs of books, list technical terms alphabetically with their definitions to aid vocabulary learning and comprehension. Boldface print is used to emphasize certain words, often identifying words included in the text's glossary where readers can look up their definitions.
- **Headings** separate sections of text and show the topic of each.
- **Subheadings** divide subject headings into smaller, more specific categories to help readers organize information.
- **Footnotes**, at the bottom of the page, give readers more information, such as citations or links.
- **Bullet points** list items separately, making facts and ideas easier to see and understand.
- A **sidebar** is a box of information to one side of the main text giving additional information, often on a more focused or in-depth example of a topic.

VISUAL FEATURES IN TEXTS

- **Illustrations** and **photographs** are pictures that visually emphasize important points in text.
- The **captions** below the illustrations explain what those images show.
- **Charts** and **tables** are visual forms of information that make something easier to understand quickly.
- **Diagrams** are drawings that show relationships or explain a process.

- **Graphs** visually show the relationships among multiple sets of information plotted along vertical and horizontal axes.
- **Maps** show geographical information visually to help readers understand the relative locations of places covered in the text.
- **Timelines** are visual graphics that show historical events in chronological order to help readers see their sequence.

Review Video: Informational Text
Visit mometrix.com/academy and enter code: 924964

Technical Language

TECHNICAL LANGUAGE

Technical language is more impersonal than literary and vernacular language. Passive voice makes the tone impersonal. For example, instead of writing, "We found this a central component of protein metabolism," scientists write, "This was found a central component of protein metabolism." While science professors have traditionally instructed students to avoid active voice because it leads to first-person ("I" and "we") usage, science editors today find passive voice dull and weak. Many journal articles combine both. Tone in technical science writing should be detached, concise, and professional. While one may normally write, "This chemical has to be available for proteins to be digested," professionals write technically, "The presence of this chemical is required for the enzyme to break the covalent bonds of proteins." The use of technical language appeals to both technical and non-technical audiences by displaying the author or speaker's understanding of the subject and suggesting their credibility regarding the message they are communicating.

TECHNICAL MATERIAL FOR NON-TECHNICAL READERS

Writing about **technical subjects** for **non-technical readers** differs from writing for colleagues because authors place more importance on delivering a critical message than on imparting the maximum technical content possible. Technical authors also must assume that non-technical audiences do not have the expertise to comprehend extremely scientific or technical messages, concepts, and terminology. They must resist the temptation to impress audiences with their scientific knowledge and expertise and remember that their primary purpose is to communicate a message that non-technical readers will understand, feel, and respond to. Non-technical and technical styles include similarities. Both should formally cite any references or other authors' work utilized in the text. Both must follow intellectual property and copyright regulations. This includes the author's protecting his or her own rights, or a public domain statement, as he or she chooses.

Review Video: Technical Passages
Visit mometrix.com/academy and enter code: 478923

NON-TECHNICAL AUDIENCES

Writers of technical or scientific material may need to write for many non-technical audiences. Some readers have no technical or scientific background, and those who do may not be in the same field as the authors. Government and corporate policymakers and budget managers need technical information they can understand for decision-making. Citizens affected by technology or science are a different audience. Non-governmental organizations can encompass many of the preceding groups. Elementary and secondary school programs also need non-technical language for presenting technical subject matter. Additionally, technical authors will need to use non-technical language when collecting consumer responses to surveys, presenting scientific or para-scientific material to the public, writing about the history of science, and writing about science and technology in developing countries.

Use of Everyday Language

Authors of technical information sometimes must write using non-technical language that readers outside their disciplinary fields can comprehend. They should use not only non-technical terms, but also normal, everyday language to accommodate readers whose native language is different than the language the text is written in. For example, instead of writing that "eustatic changes like thermal expansion are causing hazardous conditions in the littoral zone," an author would do better to write that "a rising sea level is threatening the coast." When technical terms cannot be avoided, authors should also define or explain them using non-technical language. Although authors must cite references and acknowledge their use of others' work, they should avoid the kinds of references or citations that they would use in scientific journals—unless they reinforce author messages. They should not use endnotes, footnotes, or any other complicated referential techniques because non-technical journal publishers usually do not accept them. Including high-resolution illustrations, photos, maps, or satellite images and incorporating multimedia into digital publications will enhance non-technical writing about technical subjects. Technical authors may publish using non-technical language in e-journals, trade journals, specialty newsletters, and daily newspapers.

Types of Technical Writing

Types of Printed Communication

Memo

A memo (short for *memorandum*) is a common form of written communication. There is a standard format for these documents. It is typical for there to be a **heading** at the top indicating the author, date, and recipient. In some cases, this heading will also include the author's title and the name of his or her institution. Below this information will be the **body** of the memo. These documents are typically written by and for members of the same organization. They usually contain a plan of action, a request for information on a specific topic, or a response to such a request. Memos are considered to be official documents, so they are usually written in a **formal** style. Many memos are organized with numbers or bullet points, which make it easier for the reader to identify key ideas.

Posted Announcement

People post **announcements** for all sorts of occasions. Many people are familiar with notices for lost pets, yard sales, and landscaping services. In order to be effective, these announcements need to *contain all of the information* the reader requires to act on the message. For instance, a lost pet announcement needs to include a good description of the animal and a contact number for the owner. A yard sale notice should include the address, date, and hours of the sale, as well as a brief description of the products that will be available there. When composing an announcement, it is important to consider the perspective of the **audience**—what will they need to know in order to respond to the message? Although a posted announcement can have color and decoration to attract the eye of the passerby, it must also convey the necessary information clearly.

Classified Advertisement

Classified advertisements, or **ads**, are used to sell or buy goods, to attract business, to make romantic connections, and to do countless other things. They are an inexpensive, and sometimes free, way to make a brief **pitch**. Classified ads used to be found only in newspapers or special advertising circulars, but there are now online listings as well. The style of these ads has remained basically the same. An ad usually begins with a word or phrase indicating what is being **sold** or **sought**. Then, the listing will give a brief **description** of the product or service. Because space is limited and costly in newspapers, classified ads there will often contain abbreviations for common attributes. For instance, two common abbreviations are *bk* for *black*, and *obo* for *or best offer*. Classified ads will then usually conclude by listing the **price** (or the amount the seeker is willing to pay), followed by **contact information** like a telephone number or email address.

Scale Readings of Standard Measurement Instruments

The scales used on **standard measurement instruments** are fairly easy to read with a little practice. Take the **ruler** as an example. A typical ruler has different units along each long edge. One side measures inches, and the other measures centimeters. The units are specified close to the zero reading for the ruler. Note that the ruler does not begin measuring from its outermost edge. The zero reading is a black line a tiny distance inside of the edge. On the inches side, each inch is indicated with a long black line and a number. Each half-inch is noted with a slightly shorter line. Quarter-inches are noted with still shorter lines, eighth-inches are noted with even shorter lines, and sixteenth-inches are noted with the shortest lines of all. On the centimeter side, the second-largest black lines indicate half-centimeters, and the smaller lines indicate tenths of centimeters, otherwise known as millimeters.

Visual Information in Informational Texts

Charts, Graphs, and Visuals

Tables

Tables are presented in a standard format so they will be easy to read and understand. A title is at the top, a short phrase indicating the information the table or graph intends to convey. The title of a table could be something like "Median Income for Various Education Levels" or "Price of Milk Compared to Demand." A table is composed of information laid out in vertical columns and horizontal rows. Typically, each column will have a label. If "Median Income for Various Education Levels" was placed in a table format, the two columns could be labeled "Education Level" and "Median Annual Salary." Each location on the table is called a cell, which holds a piece of information. Cells are defined by their column and row (e.g., second column, fifth row).

Median Annual Salary for Various Education Levels

Education Level	Median Annual Salary
Associate degree	$52,260
Bachelor's degree	$74,464
Master's degree	$86,372
Professional degree	$108,160
Doctoral degree	$108,316

Graphs

Like a table, a graph typically has a title at the top. This title may simply state the identities of the two axes: e.g., "Income vs. Education." However, the title may also be something more descriptive, like "A comparison of average income with level of education." In any case, bar and line graphs are laid out along two perpendicular lines, or axes. The vertical axis is called the *y*-axis, and the horizontal axis is called the *x*-axis. It is typical for the *x*-axis to be the independent variable and the

y-axis to be the dependent variable. The independent variable is the one manipulated by the researcher or creator of the graph. In the above example, the independent variable would be "education level," since the maker of the graph will define these values (associate degree, bachelor's degree, master's degree, etc.). The dependent value is not controlled by the researcher.

When selecting a graph format, it is important to consider the intention and the structure of the presentation. A bar graph is appropriate for displaying the relations between a series of distinct quantities that are on the same scale. For instance, if one wanted to display the amount of money spent on groceries during the months of a year, a bar graph would be appropriate. The vertical axis would represent values of money, and the horizontal axis would identify each month. A line graph also requires data expressed in common units, but it is better for demonstrating the general trend in that data. If the grocery expenses were plotted on a line graph instead of a bar graph, there would be more emphasis on whether the amount of money spent rose or fell over the course of the year. Whereas a bar graph is good for showing the relationships between the different values plotted, the line graph is good for showing whether the values tended to increase, decrease, or remain stable.

PIE CHART

A pie chart, also known as a circle graph, is useful for depicting how a single unit or category is divided. The standard pie chart is a circle with designated wedges. Each wedge is **proportional** in size to a part of the whole. For instance, consider Shawna, a student at City College, who uses a pie chart to represent her budget. If she spends half of her money on rent, then the pie chart will represent that amount with a line through the center of the pie. If she spends a quarter of her money on food, there will be a line extending from the edge of the circle to the center at a right angle to the line depicting rent. This illustration would make it clear that the student spends twice the amount of money on rent as she does on food.

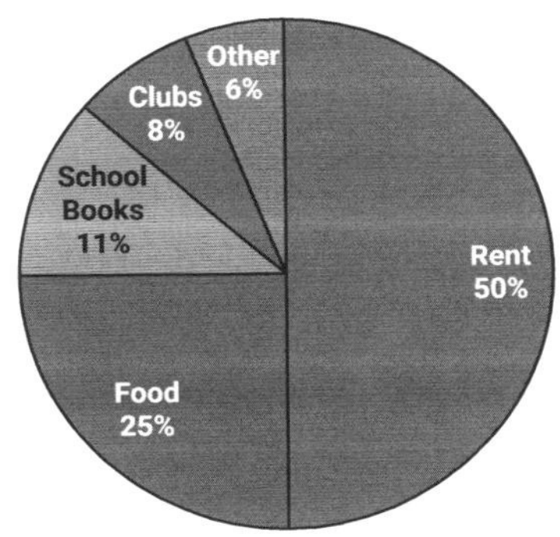

A pie chart is effective at showing how a single entity is divided into parts. They are not effective at demonstrating the relationships between parts of different wholes. For example, an unhelpful use of a pie chart would be to compare the respective amounts of state and federal spending devoted to infrastructure since these values are only meaningful in the context of the entire budget.

Bar Graph

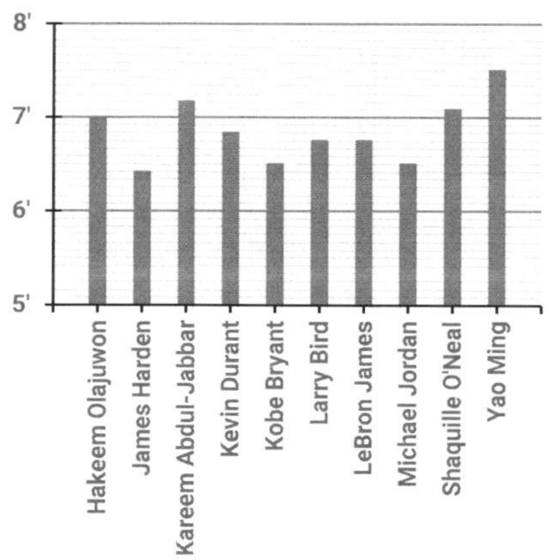

The bar graph is one of the most common visual representations of information. **Bar graphs** are used to illustrate sets of numerical **data**. The graph has a vertical axis (along which numbers are listed) and a horizontal axis (along which categories, words, or some other indicators are placed). One example of a bar graph is a depiction of the respective heights of famous basketball players: the vertical axis would contain numbers ranging from five to eight feet, and the horizontal axis would contain the names of the players. The length of the bar above the player's name would illustrate his height, and the top of the bar would stop perpendicular to the height listed along the left side. In this representation, one would see that Yao Ming is taller than Michael Jordan because Yao's bar would be higher.

Line Graph

A line graph is a type of graph that is typically used for measuring trends over time. The graph is set up along a vertical and a horizontal **axis**. The variables being measured are listed along the left side and the bottom side of the axes. Points are then plotted along the graph as they correspond with their values for each variable. For instance, consider a line graph measuring a person's income for each month of the year. If the person earned $1500 in January, there should be a point directly above January (perpendicular to the horizontal axis) and directly to the right of $1500 (perpendicular to the vertical axis). Once all of the lines are plotted, they are connected with a line from left to right. This line provides a nice visual illustration of the general **trends** of the data, if they exist. For instance, using the earlier example, if the line sloped up, then one would see that the person's income had increased over the course of the year.

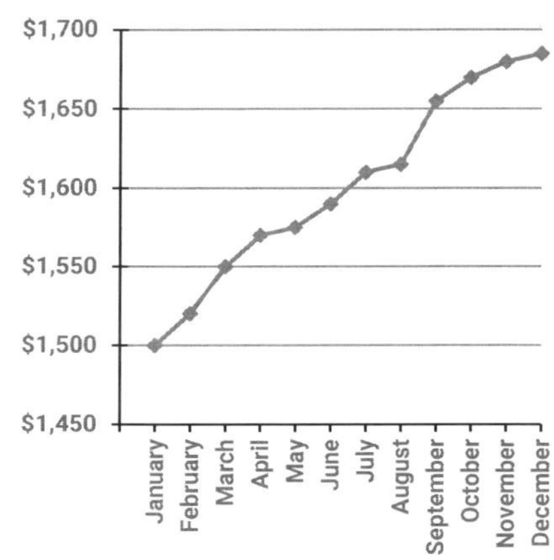

Pictographs

A **pictograph** is a graph, generally in the horizontal orientation, that uses pictures or symbols to represent the data. Each pictograph must have a key that defines the picture or symbol and gives the quantity each picture or symbol represents. Pictures or symbols on a pictograph are not always shown as whole elements. In this case, the fraction of the picture or symbol shown represents the same fraction of the quantity a whole picture or symbol stands for.

Review Video: Pictographs
Visit mometrix.com/academy and enter code: 147860

Reading Argumentative Writing

Author's Argument in Argumentative Writing

In argumentative writing, the argument is a belief, position, or opinion that the author wants to convince readers to believe as well. For the first step, readers should identify the **issue**. Some issues are controversial, meaning people disagree about them. Gun control, foreign policy, and the death penalty are all controversial issues. The next step is to determine the **author's position** on the issue. That position or viewpoint constitutes the author's argument. Readers should then identify the **author's assumptions**: things he or she accepts, believes, or takes for granted without needing proof. Inaccurate or illogical assumptions produce flawed arguments and can mislead readers. Readers should identify what kinds of **supporting evidence** the author offers, such as research results, personal observations or experiences, case studies, facts, examples, expert testimony and opinions, and comparisons. Readers should decide how relevant this support is to the argument.

Review Video: Argumentative Writing
Visit mometrix.com/academy and enter code: 561544

Evaluating an Author's Argument

The first three reader steps to **evaluate an author's argument** are to identify the **author's assumptions**, identify the **supporting evidence**, and decide **whether the evidence is relevant**. For example, if an author is not an expert on a particular topic, then that author's personal experience or opinion might not be relevant. The fourth step is to assess the **author's objectivity**. For example, consider whether the author introduces clear, understandable supporting evidence and facts to support the argument. The fifth step is evaluating whether the author's **argument is complete**. When authors give sufficient support for their arguments and also anticipate and respond effectively to opposing arguments or objections to their points, their arguments are complete. However, some authors omit information that could detract from their arguments. If instead they stated this information and refuted it, it would strengthen their arguments. The sixth step in evaluating an author's argumentative writing is to assess whether the **argument is valid**. Providing clear, logical reasoning makes an author's argument valid. Readers should ask themselves whether the author's points follow a sequence that makes sense, and whether each point leads to the next. The seventh step is to determine whether the author's **argument is credible**, meaning that it is convincing and believable. Arguments that are not valid are not credible, so step seven depends on step six. Readers should be mindful of their own biases as they evaluate and should not expect authors to conclusively prove their arguments, but rather to provide effective support and reason.

Evaluating an Author's Method of Appeal

To evaluate the effectiveness of an appeal, it is important to consider the author's purpose for writing. Any appeals an author uses in their argument must be relevant to the argument's goal. For example, a writer that argues for the reclassification of Pluto, but primarily uses appeals to emotion, will not have an effective argument. This writer should focus on using appeals to logic and support their argument with provable facts. While most arguments should include appeals to logic, emotion, and credibility, some arguments only call for one or two of these types of appeal. Evidence can support an appeal, but the evidence must be relevant to truly strengthen the appeal's effectiveness. If the writer arguing for Pluto's reclassification uses the reasons for Jupiter's classification as evidence, their argument would be weak. This information may seem relevant because it is related to the classification of planets. However, this classification is highly dependent on the size of the celestial object, and Jupiter is significantly bigger than Pluto. This use of evidence is illogical and does not support the appeal. Even when appropriate evidence and appeals are used, appeals and arguments lose their effectiveness when they create logical fallacies.

Evidence

The term **text evidence** refers to information that supports a main point or minor points and can help lead the reader to a conclusion about the text's credibility. Information used as text evidence is precise, descriptive, and factual. A main point is often followed by supporting details that provide evidence to back up a claim. For example, a passage may include the claim that winter occurs during opposite months in the Northern and Southern hemispheres. Text evidence for this claim may include examples of countries where winter occurs in opposite months. Stating that the tilt of the Earth as it rotates around the sun causes winter to occur at different times in separate hemispheres is another example of text evidence. Text evidence can come from common knowledge, but it is also valuable to include text evidence from credible, relevant outside sources.

Review Video: Textual Evidence
Visit mometrix.com/academy and enter code: 486236

Evidence that supports the thesis and additional arguments needs to be provided. Most arguments must be supported by facts or statistics. A fact is something that is known with certainty, has been verified by several independent individuals, and can be proven to be true. In addition to facts, examples and illustrations can support an argument by adding an emotional component. With this component, you persuade readers in ways that facts and statistics cannot. The emotional component is effective when used alongside objective information that can be confirmed.

Credibility

The text used to support an argument can be the argument's downfall if the text is not credible. A text is **credible**, or believable, when its author is knowledgeable and objective, or unbiased. The author's motivations for writing the text play a critical role in determining the credibility of the text and must be evaluated when assessing that credibility. Reports written about the ozone layer by an environmental scientist and a hairdresser will have a different level of credibility.

Review Video: Author Credibility
Visit mometrix.com/academy and enter code: 827257

Appeal to Emotion

Sometimes, authors will appeal to the reader's emotion in an attempt to persuade or to distract the reader from the weakness of the argument. For instance, the author may try to inspire the pity of the reader by delivering a heart-rending story. An author also might use the bandwagon approach, in which he suggests that his opinion is correct because it is held by the majority. Some authors resort to name-calling, in which insults and harsh words are delivered to the opponent in an attempt to distract. In advertising, a common appeal is the celebrity testimonial, in which a famous person endorses a product. Of course, the fact that a famous person likes something should not really mean anything to the reader. These and other emotional appeals are usually evidence of poor reasoning and a weak argument.

Review Video: Emotional Language in Literature
Visit mometrix.com/academy and enter code: 759390

Counter Arguments

When authors give both sides to the argument, they build trust with their readers. As a reader, you should start with an undecided or neutral position. If an author presents only his or her side to the argument, then they are not exhibiting credibility and are weakening their argument.

Building common ground with readers can be effective for persuading neutral, skeptical, or opposed readers. Sharing values with undecided readers can allow people to switch positions without giving up what they feel is important. People who may oppose a position need to feel that they can change their minds without betraying who they are as a person. This appeal to having an open mind can be a powerful tool in arguing a position without antagonizing other views. Objections can be countered on a point-by-point basis or in a summary paragraph. Be mindful of how an author points out flaws in counter arguments. If they are unfair to the other side of the argument, then you should lose trust with the author.

Plot and Story Structure

Plot and Story Structure

The **plot** includes the events that happen in a story and the order in which they are told to the reader. There are several types of plot structures, as stories can be told in many ways. The most common plot structure is the chronological plot, which presents the events to the reader in the same order they occur for the characters in the story. Chronological plots usually have five main parts, the **exposition**, **rising action**, the **climax**, **falling action**, and the **resolution**. This type of plot structure guides the reader through the story's events as the characters experience them and is the easiest structure to understand and identify. While this is the most common plot structure, many stories are nonlinear, which means the plot does not sequence events in the same order the characters experience them. Such stories might include elements like flashbacks that cause the story to be nonlinear.

Review Video: How to Make a Story Map
Visit mometrix.com/academy and enter code: 261719

Exposition

The **exposition** is at the beginning of the story and generally takes place before the rising action begins. The purpose of the exposition is to give the reader context for the story, which the author may do by introducing one or more characters, describing the setting or world, or explaining the events leading up to the point where the story begins. The exposition may still include events that contribute to the plot, but the **rising action** and main conflict of the story are not part of the exposition. Some narratives skip the exposition and begin the story with the beginning of the rising action, which causes the reader to learn the context as the story intensifies.

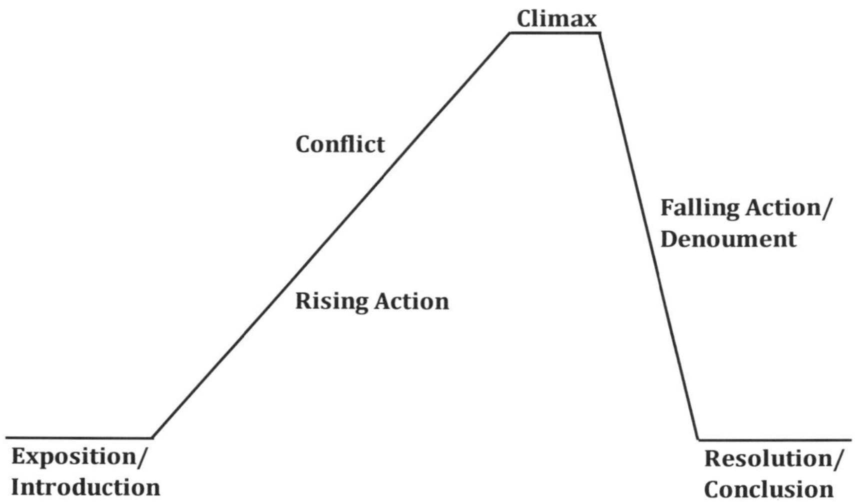

Review Video: Plot Line
Visit mometrix.com/academy and enter code: 944011

Conflict

A **conflict** is a problem to be solved. Literary plots typically include one conflict or more. Characters' attempts to resolve conflicts drive the narrative's forward movement. **Conflict resolution** is often the protagonist's primary occupation. Physical conflicts like exploring, wars, and escapes tend to make plots most suspenseful and exciting. Emotional, mental, or moral conflicts tend to make stories more personally gratifying or rewarding for many audiences. Conflicts can be external or internal. A major type of internal conflict is some inner personal battle, or **man versus self**. Major types of external conflicts include **man versus nature**, **man versus man**, and **man versus society**. Readers can identify conflicts in literary plots by identifying the protagonist and antagonist and asking why they conflict, what events develop the conflict, where the climax occurs, and how they identify with the characters.

Read the following paragraph and discuss the type of conflict present:

> Timothy was shocked out of sleep by the appearance of a bear just outside his tent. After panicking for a moment, he remembered some advice he had read in preparation for this trip: he should make noise so the bear would not be startled. As Timothy started to hum and sing, the bear wandered away.

There are three main types of conflict in literature: **man versus man**, **man versus nature**, and **man versus self**. This paragraph is an example of man versus nature. Timothy is in conflict with the bear. Even though no physical conflict like an attack exists, Timothy is pitted against the bear.

Timothy uses his knowledge to "defeat" the bear and keep himself safe. The solution to the conflict is that Timothy makes noise, the bear wanders away, and Timothy is safe.

> **Review Video: Conflict**
> Visit mometrix.com/academy and enter code: 559550
>
> **Review Video: Determining Relationships in a Story**
> Visit mometrix.com/academy and enter code: 929925

Rising Action

The **rising action** is the part of the story where conflict **intensifies**. The rising action begins with an event that prompts the main conflict of the story. This may also be called the **inciting incident**. The main conflict generally occurs between the protagonist and an antagonist, but this is not the only type of conflict that may occur in a narrative. After this event, the protagonist works to resolve the main conflict by preparing for an altercation, pursuing a goal, fleeing an antagonist, or doing some other action that will end the conflict. The rising action is composed of several additional events that increase the story's tension. Most often, other developments will occur alongside the growth of the main conflict, such as character development or the development of minor conflicts. The rising action ends with the **climax**, which is the point of highest tension in the story.

Climax

The **climax** is the event in the narrative that marks the height of the story's conflict or tension. The event that takes place at the story's climax will end the rising action and bring about the results of the main conflict. If the conflict was between a good protagonist and an evil antagonist, the climax may be a final battle between the two characters. If the conflict is an adventurer looking for heavily guarded treasure, the climax may be the adventurer's encounter with the final obstacle that protects the treasure. The climax may be made of multiple scenes, but can usually be summarized as one event. Once the conflict and climax are complete, the **falling action** begins.

Falling Action

The **falling action** shows what happens in the story between the climax and the resolution. The falling action often composes a much smaller portion of the story than the rising action does. While the climax includes the end of the main conflict, the falling action may show the results of any minor conflicts in the story. For example, if the protagonist encountered a troll on the way to find some treasure, and the troll demanded the protagonist share the treasure after retrieving it, the falling action would include the protagonist returning to share the treasure with the troll. Similarly, any unexplained major events are usually made clear during the falling action. Once all significant elements of the story are resolved or addressed, the story's resolution will occur. The **resolution** is the end of the story, which shows the final result of the plot's events and shows what life is like for the main characters once they are no longer experiencing the story's conflicts.

Resolution

The way the conflict is **resolved** depends on the type of conflict. The plot of any book starts with the lead up to the conflict, then the conflict itself, and finally the solution, or **resolution**, to the conflict. In **man versus man** conflicts, the conflict is often resolved by two parties coming to some sort of agreement or by one party triumphing over the other party. In **man versus nature** conflicts, the conflict is often resolved by man coming to some realization about some aspect of nature. In

man versus self conflicts, the conflict is often resolved by the character growing or coming to an understanding about part of himself.

THEME

A **theme** is a central idea demonstrated by a passage. Often, a theme is a lesson or moral contained in the text, but it does not have to be. It also is a unifying idea that is used throughout the text; it can take the form of a common setting, idea, symbol, design, or recurring event. A passage can have two or more themes that convey its overall idea. The theme or themes of a passage are often based on **universal themes**. They can frequently be expressed using well-known sayings about life, society, or human nature, such as "Hard work pays off" or "Good triumphs over evil." Themes are not usually stated **explicitly**. The reader must figure them out by carefully reading the passage. Themes are created through descriptive language or events in the plot. The events of a story help shape the themes of a passage.

EXAMPLE

Explain why "if you care about something, you need to take care of it" accurately describes the theme of the following excerpt.

> Luca collected baseball cards, but he wasn't very careful with them. He left them around the house. His dog liked to chew. One day, Luca and his friend Bart were looking at his collection. Then they went outside. When Luca got home, he saw his dog chewing on his cards. They were ruined.

This excerpt tells the story of a boy who is careless with his baseball cards and leaves them lying around. His dog ends up chewing them and ruining them. The lesson is that if you care about something, you need to take care of it. This is the theme, or point, of the story. Some stories have more than one theme, but this is not really true of this excerpt. The reader needs to figure out the theme based on what happens in the story. Sometimes, as in the case of fables, the theme is stated directly in the text. However, this is not usually the case.

Review Video: Themes in Literature
Visit mometrix.com/academy and enter code: 732074

Narrator's Point of View

POINT OF VIEW

Another element that impacts a text is the author's point of view. The **point of view** of a text is the perspective from which a passage is told. An author will always have a point of view about a story before he or she draws up a plot line. The author will know what events they want to take place, how they want the characters to interact, and how they want the story to resolve. An author will also have an opinion on the topic or series of events which is presented in the story that is based on their prior experience and beliefs.

The two main points of view that authors use, especially in a work of fiction, are first person and third person. If the narrator of the story is also the main character, or *protagonist*, the text is written in first-person point of view. In first person, the author writes from the perspective of *I*. Third-person point of view is probably the most common that authors use in their passages. Using third person, authors refer to each character by using *he* or *she.* In third-person omniscient, the narrator is not a character in the story and tells the story of all of the characters at the same time.

Review Video: Point of View
Visit mometrix.com/academy and enter code: 383336

First-Person Narration

First-person narratives let narrators express inner feelings and thoughts, especially when the narrator is the protagonist as Lemuel Gulliver is in Jonathan Swift's *Gulliver's Travels.* The narrator may be a close friend of the protagonist, like Dr. Watson in Sir Arthur Conan Doyle's *Sherlock Holmes.* Or, the narrator can be less involved with the main characters and plot, like Nick Carraway in F. Scott Fitzgerald's *The Great Gatsby.* When a narrator reports others' narratives, she or he is a "**frame narrator**," like the nameless narrator of Joseph Conrad's *Heart of Darkness* or Mr. Lockwood in Emily Brontë's *Wuthering Heights.* **First-person plural** is unusual but can be effective. Isaac Asimov's *I, Robot*, William Faulkner's *A Rose for Emily*, Maxim Gorky's *Twenty-Six Men and a Girl*, and Jeffrey Eugenides' *The Virgin Suicides* all use first-person plural narration. Author Kurt Vonnegut is the first-person narrator in his semi-autobiographical novel *Timequake.* Also unusual, but effective, is a **first-person omniscient** (rather than the more common third-person omniscient) narrator, like Death in Markus Zusak's *The Book Thief* and the ghost in Alice Sebold's *The Lovely Bones.*

Second-Person Narration

While **second-person** address is very commonplace in popular song lyrics, it is the least used form of narrative voice in literary works. Popular serial books of the 1980s like *Fighting Fantasy* or *Choose Your Own Adventure* employed second-person narratives. In some cases, a narrative combines both second-person and first-person voices, using the pronouns *you* and *I*. This can draw readers into the story, and it can also enable the authors to compare directly "your" and "my" feelings, thoughts, and actions. When the narrator is also a character in the story, as in Edgar Allan Poe's short story "The Tell-Tale Heart" or Jay McInerney's novel *Bright Lights, Big City,* the narrative is better defined as first-person despite it also addressing "you."

Third-Person Narration

Narration in the third person is the most prevalent type, as it allows authors the most flexibility. It is so common that readers simply assume without needing to be informed that the narrator is not a character in the story, or involved in its events. **Third-person singular** is used more frequently than **third-person plural**, though some authors have also effectively used plural. However, both singular and plural are most often included in stories according to which characters are being described. The third-person narrator may be either objective or subjective, and either omniscient or limited. **Objective third-person** narration does not include what the characters described are thinking or feeling, while **subjective third-person** narration does. The **third-person omniscient** narrator knows everything about all characters, including their thoughts and emotions, and all related places, times, and events. However, the **third-person limited** narrator may know everything about a particular character, but is limited to that character. In other words, the narrator cannot speak about anything that character does not know.

Alternating-Person Narration

Although authors more commonly write stories from one point of view, there are also instances wherein they alternate the narrative voice within the same book. For example, they may sometimes use an omniscient third-person narrator and a more intimate first-person narrator at other times. In J. K. Rowling's series of *Harry Potter* novels, she often writes in a third-person limited narrative, but sometimes changes to narration by characters other than the protagonist. George R. R. Martin's series *A Song of Ice and Fire* changes the point of view to coincide with divisions between chapters. The same technique is used by Erin Hunter (a pseudonym for several authors of the *Warriors, Seekers,* and *Survivors* book series). Authors using first-person narrative sometimes switch to third-person to describe significant action scenes, especially those where the narrator was absent or uninvolved, as Barbara Kingsolver does in her novel *The Poisonwood Bible.*

Review Video: The Narrator of a Story
Visit mometrix.com/academy and enter code: 742528

Setting, Mood, and Tone

Setting and Time Frame

A literary text has both a setting and time frame. A **setting** is the place in which the story as a whole is set. The **time frame** is the period in which the story is set. This may refer to the historical period the story takes place in or if the story takes place over a single day. Both setting and time frame are relevant to a text's meaning because they help the reader place the story in time and space. An author uses setting and time frame to anchor a text, create a mood, and enhance its meaning. This helps a reader understand why a character acts the way he does, or why certain events in the story are important. The setting impacts the **plot** and character **motivations**, while the time frame helps place the story in **chronological context**.

Example

Read the following excerpt from The Adventures of Huckleberry Finn by Mark Twain and analyze the relevance of setting to the text's meaning:

> We said there warn't no home like a raft, after all. Other places do seem so cramped up and smothery, but a raft don't. You feel mighty free and easy and comfortable on a raft.

This excerpt from *The Adventures of Huckleberry Finn* by Mark Twain reveals information about the **setting** of the book. By understanding that the main character, Huckleberry Finn, lives on a raft, the reader can place the story on a river, in this case, the Mississippi River in the South before the Civil War. The information about the setting also gives the reader clues about the **character** of Huck Finn: he clearly values independence and freedom, and he likes the outdoors. The information about the setting in the quote helps the reader to better understand the rest of the text.

Syntax and Word Choice

Authors use words and **syntax**, or sentence structure, to make their texts unique, convey their own writing style, and sometimes to make a point or emphasis. They know that word choice and syntax contribute to the reader's understanding of the text as well as to the tone and mood of a text.

Review Video: Syntax
Visit mometrix.com/academy and enter code: 242280

Mood and Tone

Mood is a story's atmosphere, or the feelings the reader gets from reading it. The way authors set the mood in writing is comparable to the way filmmakers use music to set the mood in movies. Instead of music, though, writers judiciously select descriptive words to evoke certain **moods**. The mood of a work may convey joy, anger, bitterness, hope, gloom, fear, apprehension, or any other emotion the author wants the reader to feel. In addition to vocabulary choices, authors also use figurative expressions, particular sentence structures, and choices of diction that project and reinforce the moods they want to create. Whereas mood is the reader's emotions evoked by reading what is written, **tone** is the emotions and attitudes of the writer that she or he expresses in the writing. Authors use the same literary techniques to establish tone as they do to establish mood. An author may use a humorous tone, an angry or sad tone, a sentimental or unsentimental tone, or something else entirely.

MOOD AND TONE IN THE GREAT GATSBY

To understand the difference between mood and tone, look at this excerpt from F. Scott Fitzgerald's *The Great Gatsby*. In this passage, Nick Caraway, the novel's narrator, is describing his affordable house, which sits in a neighborhood full of expensive mansions.

> "I lived at West Egg, the—well the less fashionable of the two, though this is a most superficial tag to express the bizarre and not a little sinister contrast between them. My house was at the very tip of the egg, only fifty yard from the Sound, and squeezed between two huge places that rented for twelve or fifteen thousand a season ... My own house was an eyesore, but it was a small eyesore, and it had been overlooked, so I had a view of the water, a partial view of my neighbor's lawn, and the consoling proximity of millionaires—all for eighty dollars a month."

In this description, the mood created for the reader does not match the tone created through the narrator. The mood in this passage is one of dissatisfaction and inferiority. Nick compares his home to his neighbors', saying he lives in the "less fashionable" neighborhood and that his house is "overlooked," an "eyesore," and "squeezed between two huge" mansions. He also adds that his placement allows him the "consoling proximity of millionaires." A literal reading of these details leads the reader to have negative feelings toward Nick's house and his economic inferiority to his neighbors, creating the mood.

However, Fitzgerald also conveys an opposing attitude, or tone, through Nick's description. Nick calls the distinction between the neighborhoods "superficial," showing a suspicion of the value suggested by the neighborhoods' titles, properties, and residents. Nick also undermines his critique of his own home by calling it "a small eyesore" and claiming it has "been overlooked." However, he follows these statements with a description of his surroundings, claiming that he has "a view of the water" and can see some of his wealthy neighbor's property from his home, and a comparison between the properties' rent. While the mental image created for the reader depicts a small house shoved between looming mansions, the tone suggests that Nick enjoys these qualities about his home, or at least finds it charming. He acknowledges its shortcomings, but includes the benefits of his home's unassuming appearance.

Review Video: Style, Tone, and Mood
Visit mometrix.com/academy and enter code: 416961

HISTORICAL AND SOCIAL CONTEXT

Fiction that is heavily influenced by a historical or social context cannot be comprehended as the author intended if the reader does not keep this context in mind. Many important elements of the text will be influenced by any context, including symbols, allusions, settings, and plot events. These contexts, as well as the identity of the work's author, can help to inform the reader about the author's concerns and intended meanings. For example, George Orwell published his novel *1984* in the year 1949, soon after the end of World War II. At that time, following the defeat of the Nazis, the

Cold War began between the Western Allied nations and the Eastern Soviet Communists. People were therefore concerned about the conflict between the freedoms afforded by Western democracies versus the oppression represented by Communism. Orwell had also previously fought in the Spanish Civil War against a Spanish regime that he and his fellows viewed as oppressive. From this information, readers can infer that Orwell was concerned about oppression by totalitarian governments. This informs *1984*'s story of Winston Smith's rebellion against the oppressive "Big Brother" government, of the fictional dictatorial state of Oceania, and his capture, torture, and ultimate conversion by that government. Some literary theories also seek to use historical and social contexts to reveal deeper meanings and implications in a text.

Character Development and Dialogue

CHARACTER DEVELOPMENT

When depicting characters or figures in a written text, authors generally use actions, dialogue, and descriptions as characterization techniques. Characterization can occur in both fiction and nonfiction and is used to show a character or figure's personality, demeanor, and thoughts. This helps create a more engaging experience for the reader by providing a more concrete picture of a character or figure's tendencies and features. Characterizations also gives authors the opportunity to integrate elements such as dialects, activities, attire, and attitudes into their writing.

To understand the meaning of a story, it is vital to understand the characters as the author describes them. We can look for contradictions in what a character thinks, says, and does. We can notice whether the author's observations about a character differ from what other characters in the story say about that character. A character may be dynamic, meaning they change significantly during the story, or static, meaning they remain the same from beginning to end. Characters may be two-dimensional, not fully developed, or may be well developed with characteristics that stand out vividly. Characters may also symbolize universal properties. Additionally, readers can compare and contrast characters to analyze how each one developed.

A well-known example of character development can be found in Charles Dickens's *Great Expectations*. The novel's main character, Pip, is introduced as a young boy, and he is depicted as innocent, kind, and humble. However, as Pip grows up and is confronted with the social hierarchy of Victorian England, he becomes arrogant and rejects his loved ones in pursuit of his own social advancement. Once he achieves his social goals, he realizes the merits of his former lifestyle, and lives with the wisdom he gained in both environments and life stages. Dickens shows Pip's ever-changing character through his interactions with others and his inner thoughts, which evolve as his personal values and personality shift.

DIALOGUE

Effectively written dialogue serves at least one, but usually several, purposes. It advances the story and moves the plot, develops the characters, sheds light on the work's theme or meaning, and can, often subtly, account for the passage of time not otherwise indicated. It can alter the direction that the plot is taking, typically by introducing some new conflict or changing existing ones. **Dialogue** can establish a work's narrative voice and the characters' voices and set the tone of the story or of particular characters. When fictional characters display enlightenment or realization, dialogue can give readers an understanding of what those characters have discovered and how. Dialogue can illuminate the motivations and wishes of the story's characters. By using consistent thoughts and syntax, dialogue can support character development. Skillfully created, it can also represent real-life speech rhythms in written form. Via conflicts and ensuing action, dialogue also provides drama.

Dialogue in Fiction

In fictional works, effectively written dialogue does more than just break up or interrupt sections of narrative. While **dialogue** may supply exposition for readers, it must nonetheless be believable. Dialogue should be dynamic, not static, and it should not resemble regular prose. Authors should not use dialogue to write clever similes or metaphors, or to inject their own opinions. Nor should they use dialogue at all when narrative would be better. Most importantly, dialogue should not slow the plot movement. Dialogue must seem natural, which means careful construction of phrases rather than actually duplicating natural speech, which does not necessarily translate well to the written word. Finally, all dialogue must be pertinent to the story, rather than just added conversation.

Figurative Language

Literal and Figurative Meaning

When language is used **literally**, the words mean exactly what they say and nothing more. When language is used **figuratively**, the words mean something beyond their literal meaning. For example, "The weeping willow tree has long, trailing branches and leaves" is a literal description. But "The weeping willow tree looks as if it is bending over and crying" is a figurative description—specifically, a **simile** or stated comparison. Another figurative language form is **metaphor**, or an implied comparison. A good example is the metaphor of a city, state, or city-state as a ship, and its governance as sailing that ship. Ancient Greek lyrical poet Alcaeus is credited with first using this metaphor, and ancient Greek tragedian Aeschylus then used it in *Seven Against Thebes,* and then Plato used it in the *Republic.*

Figures of Speech

A **figure of speech** is a verbal expression whose meaning is figurative rather than literal. For example, the phrase "butterflies in the stomach" does not refer to actual butterflies in a person's stomach. It is a metaphor representing the fluttery feelings experienced when a person is nervous or excited—or when one "falls in love," which does not mean physically falling. "Hitting a sales target" does not mean physically hitting a target with arrows as in archery; it is a metaphor for meeting a sales quota. "Climbing the ladder of success" metaphorically likens advancing in one's career to ascending ladder rungs. Similes, such as "light as a feather" (meaning very light, not a feather's actual weight), and hyperbole, like "I'm starving/freezing/roasting," are also figures of speech. Figures of speech are often used and crafted for emphasis, freshness of expression, or clarity.

Review Video: Figures of Speech
Visit mometrix.com/academy and enter code: 111295

Figurative Language

Figurative language extends past the literal meanings of words. It offers readers new insight into the people, things, events, and subjects covered in a work of literature. Figurative language also enables readers to feel they are sharing the authors' experiences. It can stimulate the reader's senses, make comparisons that readers find intriguing or even startling, and enable readers to view the world in different ways. When looking for figurative language, it is important to consider the context of the sentence or situation. Phrases that appear out of place or make little sense when read literally are likely instances of figurative language. Once figurative language has been recognized, context is also important to determining the type of figurative language being used and its function. For example, when a comparison is being made, a metaphor or simile is likely being used. This means the comparison may emphasize or create irony through the things being compared. Seven specific types of figurative language include: alliteration, onomatopoeia, personification, imagery, similes, metaphors, and hyperbole.

Review Video: Figurative Language
Visit mometrix.com/academy and enter code: 584902

Alliteration and Onomatopoeia

Alliteration describes a series of words beginning with the same sounds. **Onomatopoeia** uses words imitating the sounds of things they name or describe. For example, in his poem "Come Down, O Maid," Alfred Tennyson writes of "The moan of doves in immemorial elms, / And murmuring of innumerable bees." The word "moan" sounds like some sounds doves make, "murmuring" represents the sounds of bees buzzing. Onomatopoeia also includes words that are simply meant to represent sounds, such as "meow," "kaboom," and "whoosh."

Review Video: Alliteration in Everyday Expressions
Visit mometrix.com/academy and enter code: 462837

Personification

Another type of figurative language is **personification**. This is describing a non-human thing, like an animal or an object, as if it were human. The general intent of personification is to describe things in a manner that will be comprehensible to readers. When an author states that a tree *groans* in the wind, he or she does not mean that the tree is emitting a low, pained sound from a mouth. Instead, the author means that the tree is making a noise similar to a human groan. Of course, this personification establishes a tone of sadness or suffering. A different tone would be established if the author said that the tree was *swaying* or *dancing*. Alfred Tennyson's poem "The Eagle" uses all of these types of figurative language: "He clasps the crag with crooked hands." Tennyson used alliteration, repeating /k/ and /kr/ sounds. These hard-sounding consonants reinforce the imagery, giving visual and tactile impressions of the eagle.

Review Video: Personification
Visit mometrix.com/academy and enter code: 260066

Similes and Metaphors

Similes are stated comparisons using "like" or "as." Similes can be used to stimulate readers' imaginations and appeal to their senses. Because a simile includes *like* or *as,* the device creates more space between the description and the thing being described than a metaphor does. If an author says that *a house was like a shoebox*, then the tone is different than the author saying that the house *was* a shoebox. Authors will choose between a metaphor and a simile depending on their intended tone.

Similes also help compare fictional characters to well-known objects or experiences, so the reader can better relate to them. William Wordsworth's poem about "Daffodils" begins, "I wandered lonely as a cloud." This simile compares his loneliness to that of a cloud. It is also personification, giving a cloud the human quality loneliness. In his novel *Lord Jim* (1900), Joseph Conrad writes in Chapter 33, "I would have given anything for the power to soothe her frail soul, tormenting itself in its invincible ignorance like a small bird beating about the cruel wires of a cage." Conrad uses the word "like" to compare the girl's soul to a small bird. His description of the bird beating at the cage shows the similar helplessness of the girl's soul to gain freedom.

Review Video: Similes
Visit mometrix.com/academy and enter code: 642949

A **metaphor** is a type of figurative language in which the writer equates something with another thing that is not particularly similar, instead of using *like* or *as*. For instance, *the bird was an arrow arcing through the sky*. In this sentence, the arrow is serving as a metaphor for the bird. The point of a metaphor is to encourage the reader to consider the item being described in a *different way*. Let's continue with this metaphor for a flying bird. You are asked to envision the bird's flight as being similar to the arc of an arrow. So, you imagine the flight to be swift and bending. Metaphors are a way for the author to describe an item *without being direct and obvious*. This literary device is a lyrical and suggestive way of providing information. Note that the reference for a metaphor will not always be mentioned explicitly by the author. Consider the following description of a forest in winter: *Swaying skeletons reached for the sky and groaned as the wind blew through them.* In this example, the author is using *skeletons* as a metaphor for leafless trees. This metaphor creates a spooky tone while inspiring the reader's imagination.

LITERARY EXAMPLES OF METAPHOR

A **metaphor** is an implied comparison, i.e., it compares something to something else without using "like", "as", or other comparative words. For example, in "The Tyger" (1794), William Blake writes, "Tyger Tyger, burning bright, / In the forests of the night." Blake compares the tiger to a flame not by saying it is like a fire, but by simply describing it as "burning." Henry Wadsworth Longfellow's poem "O Ship of State" (1850) uses an extended metaphor by referring consistently throughout the entire poem to the state, union, or republic as a seagoing vessel, referring to its keel, mast, sail, rope, anchors, and to its braving waves, rocks, gale, tempest, and "false lights on the shore." Within the extended metaphor, Wordsworth uses a specific metaphor: "the anchors of thy hope!"

TED HUGHES' ANIMAL METAPHORS

Ted Hughes frequently used animal metaphors in his poetry. In "The Thought Fox," a model of concise, structured beauty, Hughes characterizes the poet's creative process with succinct, striking imagery of an idea entering his head like a wild fox. Repeating "loneliness" in the first two stanzas emphasizes the poet's lonely work: "Something else is alive / Beside the clock's loneliness." He treats an idea's arrival as separate from himself. Three stanzas detail in vivid images a fox's approach from the outside winter forest at starless midnight—its nose, "Cold, delicately" touching twigs and leaves; "neat" paw prints in snow; "bold" body; brilliant green eyes; and self-contained, focused progress—"Till, with a sudden sharp hot stink of fox," he metaphorically depicts poetic inspiration as the fox's physical entry into "the dark hole of the head." Hughes ends by summarizing his vision of a poet as an interior, passive idea recipient, with the outside world unchanged: "The window is starless still; the clock ticks, / The page is printed."

Review Video: Metaphors in Writing
Visit mometrix.com/academy and enter code: 133295

METONYMY

Metonymy is naming one thing with words or phrases of a closely related thing. This is similar to metaphor. However, the comparison has a close connection, unlike metaphor. An example of metonymy is to call the news media *the press*. Of course, *the press* is the machine that prints newspapers. Metonymy is a way of naming something without using the same name constantly.

Synecdoche

Synecdoche points to the whole by naming one of the parts. An example of synecdoche would be calling a construction worker a *hard hat.* Like metonymy, synecdoche is an easy way of naming something without having to overuse a name. The device allows writers to highlight pieces of the thing being described. For example, referring to businessmen as *suits* suggests professionalism and unity.

Review Video: Metonymy and Synecdoche
Visit mometrix.com/academy and enter code: 900306

Hyperbole

Hyperbole is excessive exaggeration used for humor or emphasis rather than for literal meaning. For example, in *To Kill a Mockingbird*, Harper Lee wrote, "People moved slowly then. There was no hurry, for there was nowhere to go, nothing to buy and no money to buy it with, nothing to see outside the boundaries of Maycomb County." This was not literally true; Lee exaggerates the scarcity of these things for emphasis. In "Old Times on the Mississippi," Mark Twain wrote, "I... could have hung my hat on my eyes, they stuck out so far." This is not literal, but makes his description vivid and funny. In his poem "As I Walked Out One Evening", W. H. Auden wrote, "I'll love you, dear, I'll love you / Till China and Africa meet, / And the river jumps over the mountain / And the salmon sing in the street." He used things not literally possible to emphasize the duration of his love.

Understatement

Understatement is the opposite of hyperbole. This device discounts or downplays something. Think about someone who climbs Mount Everest. Then, they say that the journey was *a little stroll.* As with other types of figurative language, understatement has a range of uses. The device may show self-defeat or modesty as in the Mount Everest example. However, some may think of understatement as false modesty (i.e., an attempt to bring attention to you or a situation). For example, a woman is praised on her diamond engagement ring. The woman says, *Oh, this little thing?* Her understatement might be heard as stuck-up or unfeeling.

Review Video: Hyperbole and Understatement
Visit mometrix.com/academy and enter code: 308470

Literary Devices

Literary Irony

In literature, irony demonstrates the opposite of what is said or done. The three types of irony are **verbal irony**, **situational irony**, and **dramatic irony**. Verbal irony uses words opposite to the meaning. Sarcasm may use verbal irony. One common example is describing something that is confusing as "clear as mud." For example, in his 1986 movie *Hannah and Her Sisters,* author, director, and actor Woody Allen says to his character's date, "I had a great evening; it was like the Nuremburg Trials." Notice these employ similes. In situational irony, what happens contrasts with what was expected. O. Henry's short story *The Gift of the Magi* uses situational irony: a husband and wife each sacrifice their most prized possession to buy each other a Christmas present. The irony is that she sells her long hair to buy him a watch fob, while he sells his heirloom pocket-watch to buy her the jeweled combs for her hair she had long wanted; in the end, neither of them can use their gifts. In dramatic irony, narrative informs audiences of more than its characters know. For example, in *Romeo and Juliet,* the audience is made aware that Juliet is only asleep, while Romeo believes her to be dead, which then leads to Romeo's death.

Review Video: Irony
Visit mometrix.com/academy and enter code: 374204

Idioms

Idioms create comparisons, and often take the form of similes or metaphors. Idioms are always phrases and are understood to have a meaning that is different from its individual words' literal meaning. For example, "break a leg" is a common idiom that is used to wish someone luck or tell them to perform well. Literally, the phrase "break a leg" means to injure a person's leg, but the phrase takes on a different meaning when used as an idiom. Another example is "call it a day," which means to temporarily stop working on a task, or find a stopping point, rather than literally referring to something as "a day." Many idioms are associated with a region or group. For example, an idiom commonly used in the American South is "'til the cows come home." This phrase is often used to indicate that something will take or may last for a very long time, but not that it will literally last until the cows return to where they reside.

Allusion

An allusion is an uncited but recognizable reference to something else. Authors use language to make allusions to places, events, artwork, and other books in order to make their own text richer. For example, an author may allude to a very important text in order to make his own text seem more important. Martin Luther King, Jr. started his "I Have a Dream" speech by saying "Five score years ago…" This is a clear allusion to President Abraham Lincoln's "Gettysburg Address" and served to remind people of the significance of the event. An author may allude to a place to ground his text or make a cultural reference to make readers feel included. There are many reasons that authors make allusions.

Review Video: Allusions
Visit mometrix.com/academy and enter code: 294065

Comic Relief

Comic relief is the use of comedy by an author to break up a dramatic or tragic scene and infuse it with a bit of **lightheartedness**. In William Shakespeare's *Hamlet*, two gravediggers digging the grave for Ophelia share a joke while they work. The death and burial of Ophelia are tragic moments that directly follow each other. Shakespeare uses an instance of comedy to break up the tragedy and give his audience a bit of a break from the tragic drama. Authors sometimes use comic relief so that their work will be less depressing; other times they use it to create irony or contrast between the darkness of the situation and the lightness of the joke. Often, authors will use comedy to parallel what is happening in the tragic scenes.

Review Video: Comic Relief
Visit mometrix.com/academy and enter code: 779604

FORESHADOWING

Foreshadowing is a device authors use to give readers **hints** about events that will take place later in a story. Foreshadowing most often takes place through a character's dialogue or actions. Sometimes the character will know what is going to happen and will purposefully allude to future events. For example, consider a protagonist who is about to embark on a journey through the woods. Just before the protagonist begins the trip, another character says, "Be careful, you never know what could be out in those woods!" This alerts the reader that the woods may be dangerous and prompts the reader to expect something to attack the protagonist in the woods. This is an example of foreshadowing through warning. Alternatively, a character may unknowingly foreshadow later events. For example, consider a story where a brother and sister run through their house and knock over a vase and break it. The brother says, "Don't worry, we'll clean it up! Mom will never know!" However, the reader knows that their mother will most likely find out what they have done, so the reader expects the siblings to later get in trouble for running, breaking the vase, and hiding it from their mother.

SYMBOLISM

Symbolism describes an author's use of a **symbol**, an element of the story that **represents** something else. Symbols can impact stories in many ways, including deepening the meaning of a story or its elements, comparing a story to another work, or foreshadowing later events in a story. Symbols can be objects, characters, colors, numbers, or anything else the author establishes as a symbol. Symbols can be clearly established through direct comparison or repetition, but they can also be established subtly or gradually over a large portion of the story. Another form of symbolism is **allusion**, which is when something in a story is used to prompt the reader to think about another work. Many well-known works use **Biblical allusions**, which are allusions to events or details in the Bible that inform a work or an element within it.

Chapter Quiz

Ready to see how well you retained what you just read? Scan the QR code to go directly to the chapter quiz interface for this study guide. If you're using a computer, simply visit the online resources page at **mometrix.com/resources719/pnat** and click the Chapter Quizzes link.

Numerical Ability

Number Basics

Classifications of Numbers

Numbers are the basic building blocks of mathematics. Specific features of numbers are identified by the following terms:

Integer – any positive or negative whole number, including zero. Integers do not include fractions $\left(\frac{1}{3}\right)$, decimals (0.56), or mixed numbers $\left(7\frac{3}{4}\right)$.

Prime number – any whole number greater than 1 that has only two factors, itself and 1; that is, a number that can be divided evenly only by 1 and itself.

Composite number – any whole number greater than 1 that has more than two different factors; in other words, any whole number that is not a prime number. For example: The composite number 8 has the factors of 1, 2, 4, and 8.

Even number – any integer that can be divided by 2 without leaving a remainder. For example: 2, 4, 6, 8, and so on.

Odd number – any integer that cannot be divided evenly by 2. For example: 3, 5, 7, 9, and so on.

Decimal number – any number that uses a decimal point to show the part of the number that is less than one. Example: 1.234.

Decimal point – a symbol used to separate the ones place from the tenths place in decimals or dollars from cents in currency.

Decimal place – the position of a number to the right of the decimal point. In the decimal 0.123, the 1 is in the first place to the right of the decimal point, indicating tenths; the 2 is in the second place, indicating hundredths; and the 3 is in the third place, indicating thousandths.

The **decimal**, or base 10, system is a number system that uses ten different digits (0, 1, 2, 3, 4, 5, 6, 7, 8, 9). An example of a number system that uses something other than ten digits is the **binary**, or base 2, number system, used by computers, which uses only the numbers 0 and 1. It is thought that the decimal system originated because people had only their 10 fingers for counting.

Rational numbers include all integers, decimals, and fractions. Any terminating or repeating decimal number is a rational number.

Irrational numbers cannot be written as fractions or decimals because the number of decimal places is infinite and there is no recurring pattern of digits within the number. For example, pi (π) begins with 3.141592 and continues without terminating or repeating, so pi is an irrational number.

Real numbers are the set of all rational and irrational numbers.

Review Video: Classification of Numbers
Visit mometrix.com/academy and enter code: 461071

Review Video: Prime and Composite Numbers
Visit mometrix.com/academy and enter code: 565581

NUMBERS IN WORD FORM AND PLACE VALUE

When writing numbers out in word form or translating word form to numbers, it is essential to understand how a place value system works. In the decimal or base-10 system, each digit of a number represents how many of the corresponding place value—a specific factor of 10—are contained in the number being represented. To make reading numbers easier, every three digits to the left of the decimal place is preceded by a comma. The following table demonstrates some of the place values:

Power of 10	10^3	10^2	10^1	10^0	10^{-1}	10^{-2}	10^{-3}
Value	1,000	100	10	1	0.1	0.01	0.001
Place	thousands	hundreds	tens	ones	tenths	hundredths	thousandths

For example, consider the number 4,546.09, which can be separated into each place value like this:

4: thousands
5: hundreds
4: tens
6: ones
0: tenths
9: hundredths

This number in word form would be *four thousand five hundred forty-six and nine hundredths.*

Review Video: Place Value
Visit mometrix.com/academy and enter code: 205433

Number Lines

A number line is a graph to see the distance between numbers. Basically, this graph shows the relationship between numbers. So a number line may have a point for zero and may show negative numbers on the left side of the line. Any positive numbers are placed on the right side of the line. For example, consider the points labeled on the following number line:

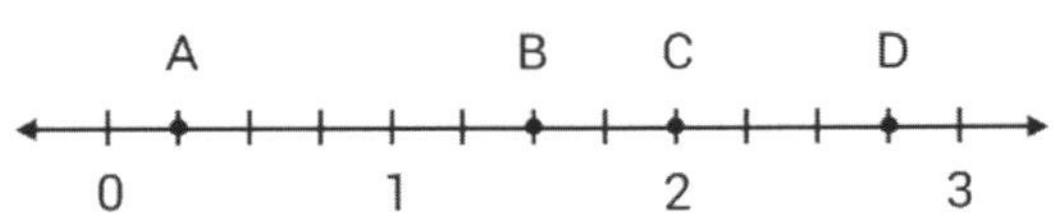

We can use the dashed lines on the number line to identify each point. Each dashed line between two whole numbers is $\frac{1}{4}$. The line halfway between two numbers is $\frac{1}{2}$.

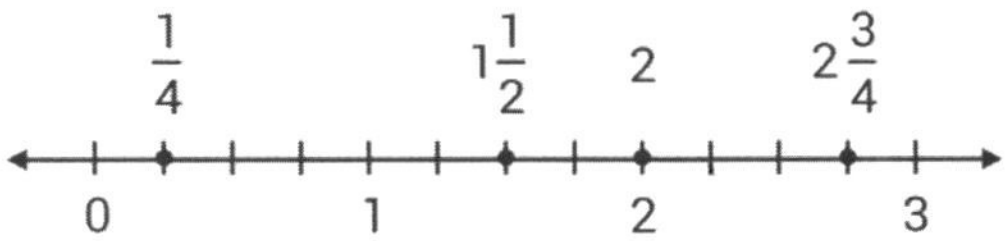

Review Video: The Number Line
Visit mometrix.com/academy and enter code: 816439

Comparing Numbers

Inequality Notation

The symbols $<$ and $>$ mean "is less than" and "is greater than," respectively. For instance, $3 < 5$ means "3 is less than 5," and $7 > 4$ means "7 is greater than 4." Statements like $3 < 5$ and $7 > 4$ are **inequalities**, and the symbols $<$ and $>$ are **inequality symbols**.

Whole Numbers and Decimal Numbers

To compare whole or decimal numbers, we look at the most significant place (the leftmost digit) at which they differ. The number with the larger digit in that place is larger. For instance, $0.3\underline{8}74$ and $0.3\underline{9}$ differ in the hundredths place (underlined). Since 8 is smaller than 9, we see $0.3874 < 0.39$. This is clearer if we make the decimals equal in length by writing extra zeroes: $0.3874 < 0.3900$. Similarly, $2\underline{3}.984 < 2\underline{5}.112$ because 3 is smaller than 5, or 23 is smaller than 25.

Fractions

If fractions have the same denominator, the fraction with the larger numerator is larger. For instance, $\frac{2}{7} < \frac{5}{7}$ since $2 < 5$. We compare fractions with different denominators by finding a common denominator. When comparing the fractions with a common denominator we only compare the numerator, so as a shortcut, we can multiply each numerator by the denominator of the other fraction. The numerator that produces the larger product belongs to the larger fraction. For example, to compare $\frac{7}{8}$ and $\frac{5}{6}$, we note that $7 \cdot 6 = 42$ is larger than $5 \cdot 8 = 40$. Since the numerator 7 produces the larger product, we see $\frac{7}{8} > \frac{5}{6}$. We can also compare fractions by converting them to decimals. For instance, since $\frac{3}{4} = 0.75$ and $\frac{4}{5} = 0.8$ and $0.75 < 0.8$, we conclude $\frac{3}{4} < \frac{4}{5}$.

Mixed Numbers

To compare mixed numbers we compare their whole number parts. If those are equal, then we compare their fractional parts. For instance, $5\frac{3}{8} > 4\frac{7}{8}$ because $5 > 4$, but $3\frac{5}{9} < 3\frac{8}{9}$ because $\frac{5}{9} < \frac{8}{9}$.

Square Roots

To compare square roots, we convert them to decimals, usually with a calculator. To compare two square roots, we compare their radicands. For instance, $\sqrt{11} < \sqrt{14}$ because $11 < 14$.

Negative Numbers

A negative number is always less than a positive number. Two negative numbers compare in the reverse order of their opposites. For instance, $-6 < -2$ (that is, -6 is smaller, more negative, than -2) because $6 > 2$.

Rounding and Estimation

Rounding is reducing the digits in a number while still trying to keep the value similar. The result will be less accurate but in a simpler form and easier to use. Whole numbers can be rounded to the nearest ten, hundred, or thousand, for instance.

To round a number, we make it a little smaller (rounding down) or a little larger (rounding up) to get a number that ends in zeros. We specify the number of zeros by naming the last place that we will not "zero out." For example, to round 8,3̲27 to the nearest hundred, we round down to 8,3̲00, zeroing out every digit to the right of the hundreds place. To round 4̲,728 to the nearest thousand, we round up to 5̲,000, increasing the thousands digit by one (to make the number larger) and zeroing out every digit to the right of the thousands place.

We decide whether to round down or up by looking at the first digit we are going to zero out. If it is less than 5 (namely, 0, 1, 2, 3, or 4) we round down. If it is greater than or equal to 5 (namely, 5, 6, 7, 8, or 9) we round up by adding 1 to the place we are rounding to. So, rounding 8,3̲27 to the nearest hundred, we round down to 8,3̲00 because the tens digit, 2, is less than 5. And rounding 4̲,728 to the nearest thousand, we round up to 5̲,000, increasing the thousands digit by 1, because the hundreds digit, 7, is greater than or equal to 5.

This even works with decimals. For example, rounding 39.7̲426 to the nearest tenth, we round down to 39.7̲000 (or simply 39.7̲) because the hundredths digit, 4, is less than 5. And rounding 0.019̲823 to the nearest thousandth, we round up to 0.020̲000 (or simply 0.02) by increasing the thousandths digit by 1, because the ten-thousandths digit, 8, is greater than or equal to 5.

When you are asked to estimate the solution to a problem, you will need to provide only an approximate figure or **estimation** for your answer. In this situation, you will need to round each number in the calculation to the level indicated (nearest hundred, nearest thousand, etc.) or to a level that makes sense for the numbers involved. When estimating a sum **all numbers must be rounded to the same level**. You cannot round one number to the nearest thousand while rounding another to the nearest hundred.

For instance, suppose you are considering buying four pieces of equipment for your home office. Their prices are \$485, \$1,217, \$750, and \$643. To estimate their total cost, you might round each price to the nearest hundred and add the rounded figures, getting an estimate of $\$500 + \$1{,}200 + \$800 + \$600 = \$3{,}100$. By estimating instead of making an exact calculation, you give up a little accuracy to get a simpler calculation.

Review Video: Rounding and Estimation
Visit mometrix.com/academy and enter code: 126243

Absolute Value

A precursor to working with negative numbers is understanding what **absolute values** are. A number's absolute value is simply the distance away from zero a number is on the number line. The absolute value of a number is always positive and is written $|x|$. For example, the absolute value of

3, written as $|3|$, is 3 because the distance between 0 and 3 on a number line is three units. Likewise, the absolute value of –3, written as $|-3|$, is 3 because the distance between 0 and –3 on a number line is three units. So $|3| = |-3|$.

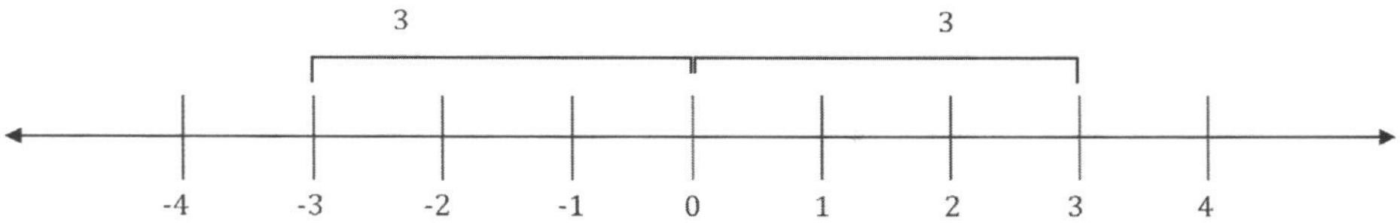

Review Video: Absolute Value
Visit mometrix.com/academy and enter code: 314669

Operations

An **operation** is simply a mathematical process that takes some value(s) as input(s) and produces an output. Elementary operations are often written in the following form: *value operation value*. For instance, in the expression $1 + 2$ the values are 1 and 2 and the operation is addition. Performing the operation gives the output of 3. In this way we can say that $1 + 2$ and 3 are equal, or $1 + 2 = 3$.

Addition

Addition increases the value of one quantity by the value of another quantity (both called **addends**). Example: $2 + 4 = 6$ or $8 + 9 = 17$. The result is called the **sum**. With addition, the order does not matter, $4 + 2 = 2 + 4$.

When adding signed numbers, if the signs are the same simply add the absolute values of the addends and apply the original sign to the sum. For example, $(+4) + (+8) = +12$ and $(-4) + (-8) = -12$. When the original signs are different, take the absolute values of the addends and subtract the smaller value from the larger value, then apply the original sign of the larger value to the difference. Example: $(+4) + (-8) = -4$ and $(-4) + (+8) = +4$.

Subtraction

Subtraction is the opposite operation to addition; it decreases the value of one quantity (the **minuend**) by the value of another quantity (the **subtrahend**). For example, $6 - 4 = 2$ or $17 - 8 = 9$. The result is called the **difference**. Note that with subtraction, the order does matter, $6 - 4 \neq 4 - 6$.

For subtracting signed numbers, change the sign of the subtrahend and then follow the same rules used for addition. Example: $(+4) - (+8) = (+4) + (-8) = -4$

Multiplication

Multiplication can be thought of as repeated addition. One number (the **multiplier**) indicates how many times to add the other number (the **multiplicand**) to itself. Example: $3 \times 2 = 2 + 2 + 2 = 6$. With multiplication, the order does not matter, $2 \times 3 = 3 \times 2$ or $3 + 3 = 2 + 2 + 2$, either way the result (the **product**) is the same.

If the signs are the same, the product is positive when multiplying signed numbers. Example: $(+4) \times (+8) = +32$ and $(-4) \times (-8) = +32$. If the signs are opposite, the product is negative. Example: $(+4) \times (-8) = -32$ and $(-4) \times (+8) = -32$. When more than two factors are multiplied together, the sign of the product is determined by how many negative factors are present. If there are an odd number of negative factors then the product is negative, whereas an even number of negative factors indicates a positive product. Example: $(+4) \times (-8) \times (-2) = +64$ and $(-4) \times (-8) \times (-2) = -64$.

Division

Division is the opposite operation to multiplication; one number (the **divisor**) tells us how many parts to divide the other number (the **dividend**) into. The result of division is called the **quotient**. Example: $20 \div 4 = 5$. If 20 is split into 4 equal parts, each part is 5. With division, the order of the numbers does matter, $20 \div 4 \neq 4 \div 20$.

The rules for dividing signed numbers are similar to multiplying signed numbers. If the dividend and divisor have the same sign, the quotient is positive. If the dividend and divisor have opposite signs, the quotient is negative. Example: $(-4) \div (+8) = -0.5$.

Review Video: Mathematical Operations
Visit mometrix.com/academy and enter code: 208095

Parentheses

Parentheses are used to designate which operations should be done first when there are multiple operations. Example: $4 - (2 + 1) = 1$; the parentheses tell us that we must add 2 and 1, and then subtract the sum from 4, rather than subtracting 2 from 4 and then adding 1 (this would give us an answer of 3).

Review Video: Mathematical Parentheses
Visit mometrix.com/academy and enter code: 978600

Exponents

An **exponent** is a superscript number placed next to another number at the top right. It indicates how many times the base number is to be multiplied by itself. Exponents provide a shorthand way to write what would be a longer mathematical expression. Example: $2^4 = 2 \times 2 \times 2 \times 2$. A number with an exponent of 2 is said to be "squared," while a number with an exponent of 3 is said to be "cubed." The value of a number raised to an exponent is called its power. So 8^4 is read as "8 to the 4th power," or "8 raised to the power of 4."

Review Video: Exponents
Visit mometrix.com/academy and enter code: 600998

Roots

A **root**, such as a square root, is another way of writing a fractional exponent. Instead of using a superscript, roots use the radical symbol ($\sqrt{}$) to indicate the operation. A radical will have a number underneath the bar, and may sometimes have a number in the upper left: $\sqrt[n]{a}$, read as "the nth root of a." The relationship between radical notation and exponent notation can be described by this equation:

$$\sqrt[n]{a} = a^{\frac{1}{n}}$$

The two special cases of $n = 2$ and $n = 3$ are called square roots and cube roots. If there is no number to the upper left, the radical is understood to be a square root ($n = 2$). Nearly all of the roots you encounter will be square roots. A square root is the same as a number raised to the one-half power. When we say that a is the square root of b ($a = \sqrt{b}$), we mean that a multiplied by itself equals b: ($a \times a = b$).

A **perfect square** is a number that has an integer for its square root. There are 10 perfect squares from 1 to 100: 1, 4, 9, 16, 25, 36, 49, 64, 81, 100 (the squares of integers 1 through 10).

Review Video: Roots
Visit mometrix.com/academy and enter code: 795655

Review Video: Perfect Squares and Square Roots
Visit mometrix.com/academy and enter code: 648063

Word Problems and Mathematical Symbols

When working on word problems, you must be able to translate verbal expressions or "math words" into math symbols. This chart contains several "math words" and their appropriate symbols:

Phrase	Symbol
equal, is, was, will be, has, costs, gets to, is the same as, becomes	$=$
times, of, multiplied by, product of, twice, doubles, halves, triples	$\times$
divided by, per, ratio of/to, out of	$\div$
plus, added to, sum, combined, and, more than, totals of	$+$
subtracted from, less than, decreased by, minus, difference between	$-$
what, how much, original value, how many, a number, a variable	x, n, etc.

Review Video: Understanding Word Problems
Visit mometrix.com/academy and enter code: 499199

Examples of Translated Mathematical Phrases

- The phrase four more than twice a number can be written algebraically as $2x + 4$.
- The phrase half a number decreased by six can be written algebraically as $\frac{1}{2}x - 6$.
- The phrase the sum of a number and the product of five and that number can be written algebraically as $x + 5x$.
- You may see a test question that says, "Olivia is constructing a bookcase from seven boards. Two of them are for vertical supports and five are for shelves. The height of the bookcase is twice the width of the bookcase. If the seven boards total 36 feet in length, what will be the height of Olivia's bookcase?" You would need to make a sketch and then create the equation to determine the width of the shelves. The height can be represented as double the width. (If x represents the width of the shelves in feet, then the height of the bookcase is $2x$. Since the seven boards total 36 feet, $2x + 2x + x + x + x + x + x = 36$ or $9x = 36$; $x = 4$. The height is twice the width, or 8 feet.)

Subtraction with Regrouping

A great way to make use of some of the features built into the decimal system would be regrouping when attempting longform subtraction operations. When subtracting within a place value, sometimes the minuend is smaller than the subtrahend; **regrouping** enables you to 'borrow' a unit from a place value to the left in order to get a positive difference. For example, consider subtracting 189 from 525 with regrouping.

First, set up the subtraction problem in vertical form:

$$\begin{array}{r} 525 \\ -\ 189 \\ \hline \end{array}$$

Notice that the numbers in the ones and tens columns of 525 are smaller than the numbers in the ones and tens columns of 189. This means you will need to use regrouping to perform subtraction:

$$\begin{array}{cccc} & 5 & 2 & 5 \\ - & 1 & 8 & 9 \\ \hline \end{array}$$

To subtract 9 from 5 in the ones column you will need to borrow from the 2 in the tens column:

$$\begin{array}{cccc} & 5 & 1 & 15 \\ - & 1 & 8 & 9 \\ \hline & & & 6 \end{array}$$

Next, to subtract 8 from 1 in the tens column you will need to borrow from the 5 in the hundreds column:

$$\begin{array}{cccc} & 4 & 11 & 15 \\ - & 1 & 8 & 9 \\ \hline & & 3 & 6 \end{array}$$

Last, subtract the 1 from the 4 in the hundreds column:

$$\begin{array}{cccc} & 4 & 11 & 15 \\ - & 1 & 8 & 9 \\ \hline & 3 & 3 & 6 \end{array}$$

Review Video: Subtracting Large Numbers
Visit mometrix.com/academy and enter code: 603350

Order of Operations

The **order of operations** is a set of rules that dictates the order in which we must perform each operation in an expression so that we will evaluate it accurately. If we have an expression that includes multiple different operations, the order of operations tells us which operations to do first. The most common mnemonic for the order of operations is **PEMDAS**, or "Please Excuse My Dear Aunt Sally." PEMDAS stands for parentheses, exponents, multiplication, division, addition, and subtraction. It is important to understand that multiplication and division have equal precedence, as do addition and subtraction, so those pairs of operations are simply worked from left to right in order.

For example, evaluating the expression $5 + 20 \div 4 \times (2 + 3)^2 - 6$ using the correct order of operations would be done like this:

- **P:** Perform the operations inside the parentheses: $(2 + 3) = 5$
- **E:** Simplify the exponents: $(5)^2 = 5 \times 5 = 25$
    - The expression now looks like this: $5 + 20 \div 4 \times 25 - 6$
- **MD:** Perform multiplication and division from left to right: $20 \div 4 = 5$; then $5 \times 25 = 125$
    - The expression now looks like this: $5 + 125 - 6$
- **AS:** Perform addition and subtraction from left to right: $5 + 125 = 130$; then $130 - 6 = 124$

Review Video: Order of Operations
Visit mometrix.com/academy and enter code: 259675

Properties of Operations

The Commutative Property

The commutative property applies to addition and multiplication and states that these operations can be completed in any order. The **commutative property of addition** states that numbers and terms can be added together in any order to still get the same value. For example, $3 + 4 = 7$ and $4 + 3 = 7$. Also, we can use the commutative property of addition to show that $3x + 4 + 2^2$ is equivalent to $4 + 3x + 2^2$ and $2^2 + 4 + 3x$. When adding terms, you can add in any order and get the same value.

The **commutative property of multiplication** states that numbers and terms can be multiplied in any order to get the same value. For example, 12×3 is equivalent to 3×12. Additionally, we can use the commutative property of multiplication to assume that $(5 + 3) \times (36 - 6)$ is equivalent to $(36 - 6) \times (5 + 3)$. You can multiply terms in any order and still get the same value.

The Associative Property

The **associative property of addition** states that if three or more terms are being added together, the value is the same regardless of the groupings.

For example, given the expression $3 + 4 + 6$, these terms can be grouped and added in any form. $3 + 4 + 6$ is equivalent to $(3 + 4) + 6$ and is also equivalent to $3 + (4 + 6)$. This can be applied to write equivalent expressions in a variety of ways.

For example, suppose we are given the expression $5 + (y + 2) + 4$. We can generate equivalent expressions knowing the associative property. Knowing that when three or more terms are added, the grouping is irrelevant, we can say that this expression is equivalent to $5 + y + (2 + 4)$, and it is equivalent to $(5 + y) + (2 + 4)$. It is even equivalent to $5 + y + 2 + 4$.

The **associative property of multiplication** states that if three or more terms are being multiplied together, the value is the same regardless of the grouping. We can use this property to identify and generate equivalent expressions.

For example, given the expression $2 \times 7 \times 3$, these terms can be grouped in any way and still get the same value. $2 \times 7 \times 3$ is equivalent to $(2 \times 7) \times 3$ or $2 \times (7 \times 3)$.

The Identity Property

The **identity property of multiplication** states that when a number is multiplied by 1, you get the same number. That is, anything multiplied by 1 is itself. For example, $2 \times 1 = 2$, or $1 \times -36 = -36$. Using the identity property of multiplication, we can identify and generate equivalent expressions. Let's say that we are given the expression $15 - (3 \times 4)$. We can generate equivalent expressions using the identity property. One equivalent expression example would be $(15 \times 1) - (3 \times 4)$. Another example would be $15 - (1 \times 3 \times 4)$. We can say these expressions are equivalent because the identity property of multiplication states that we can multiply any portion of an expression by 1 to get the same value.

The **identity property of addition** states that when 0 is added to a number, you get the same number. For example, $2 + 0 = 2$, or $0 + -3 = -3$. We can also use this property to identify and generate equivalent expressions. For example, if we are given the expression $2 \times (1 + 2)$, we could write the equivalent expressions $2 \times (0 + 1 + 2)$ or $(2 + 0) \times (1 + 2)$.

The Inverse Property

The **inverse property of addition** states that the sum of a number and its opposite is always equal to 0. Remember, the opposite of a number is a number that is opposite on the number line from zero, or the same number with the opposite sign. For example, −4 is opposite to 4, and 1,726.9 is opposite to −1,726.9. So, the inverse property of addition states that if you add opposite numbers, their sum is zero. For example, $5 + (-5) = 0$ and $-5 + 5 = 0$.

The **inverse property of multiplication** states that a number multiplied by its reciprocal is always equal to 1. The **reciprocal** of a number is its "flipped" fraction. For example, the reciprocal of 5 is $\frac{1}{5}$, or the reciprocal of $\frac{2}{3}$ is $\frac{3}{2}$. The inverse property of multiplication can be applied for these values, $5 \times \frac{1}{5} = 1$ and $\frac{2}{3} \times \frac{3}{2} = 1$. This is because when you multiply across, you get a fraction that is equal to 1.

$$\frac{2}{3} \times \frac{3}{2} = \frac{6}{6} = 1$$

The Distributive Property

The **distributive property** explains how multiplication and addition interact. It says that when multiplying one number by the sum of two other numbers, the same result can also be obtained by multiplying the one number by each of the numbers individually and then adding the products. For example, to multiply 2 by the sum of 7 and 3, the direct approach says, "the sum of 7 and 3 is 10, and 2 times 10 is 20." This would be expressed as $2 \times (7 + 3) = 2 \times 10 = 20$. On the other hand, the distributive property states that the same answer can be achieved by multiplying each number inside the parentheses and adding the products. That is, "the product of 2 and 7 is 14, the product of 2 and 3 is 6, and the sum of 14 and 6 is 20." This would be expressed as $2 \times (7 + 3) = 2 \times 7 + 2 \times 3 = 14 + 6 = 20$, and it is demonstrated below.

$$2 \times (7 + 3) = 2 \times 7 + 2 \times 3$$

This same concept can be used when multiplying a number by the difference of two numbers. For example, $5 \times (10 - 4) = 5 \times 10 - 5 \times 4$. Since $5 \times 10 = 50$ and $5 \times 4 = 20$, the result is $50 - 20 =$

30. This answer can be checked by subtracting inside the parentheses first and then multiplying: $5 \times (10 - 4) = 5 \times 6 = 30$.

Review Video: Commutative, Associative, and Distributive Properties
Visit mometrix.com/academy and enter code: 483176

Properties of Exponents

The properties of exponents are as follows:

Property	Description
$a^1 = a$	Any number to the power of 1 is equal to itself
$1^n = 1$	The number 1 raised to any power is equal to 1
$a^0 = 1$	Any number raised to the power of 0 is equal to 1
$a^n \times a^m = a^{n+m}$	Add exponents to multiply powers of the same base number
$a^n \div a^m = a^{n-m}$	Subtract exponents to divide powers of the same base number
$(a^n)^m = a^{n \times m}$	When a power is raised to a power, the exponents are multiplied
$(a \times b)^n = a^n \times b^n$ $(a \div b)^n = a^n \div b^n$	Multiplication and division operations inside parentheses can be raised to a power. This is the same as each term being raised to that power.
$a^{-n} = \frac{1}{a^n}$	A negative exponent is the same as the reciprocal of a positive exponent

Note that exponents do not have to be integers. Fractional or decimal exponents follow all the rules above as well. Example: $5^{\frac{1}{4}} \times 5^{\frac{3}{4}} = 5^{\frac{1}{4}+\frac{3}{4}} = 5^1 = 5$.

Review Video: Properties of Exponents
Visit mometrix.com/academy and enter code: 532558

Scientific Notation

Scientific notation is a way of writing large numbers in a shorter form. The form $a \times 10^n$ is used in scientific notation, where a is greater than or equal to 1 but less than 10, and n is the number of places the decimal must move to get from the original number to a. Example: The number 230,400,000 is cumbersome to write. To write the value in scientific notation, place a decimal point between the first and second numbers, and include all digits through the last non-zero digit ($a = 2.304$). To find the appropriate power of 10, count the number of places the decimal point had to move ($n = 8$). The number is positive if the decimal moved to the left, and negative if it moved to the right. We can then write 230,400,000 as 2.304×10^8. If we look instead at the number 0.00002304, we have the same value for a, but this time the decimal moved 5 places to the right ($n = -5$). Thus, 0.00002304 can be written as 2.304×10^{-5}. Using this notation makes it simple to compare very large or very small numbers. By comparing exponents, it is easy to see that 3.28×10^4 is smaller than 1.51×10^5, because 4 is less than 5.

Review Video: Scientific Notation
Visit mometrix.com/academy and enter code: 976454

Factors and Multiples

Factors and Greatest Common Factor

A whole number a is a **factor** (or **divisor**) of a whole number b if a divides b evenly. In other words, a is a factor of b if the quotient $b \div a$ is a whole number with a remainder of 0. For instance, 3 is a factor of 12 because $12 \div 3 = 4$ with no remainder. Another way to say this is that a is a factor of b if we can multiply a by another whole number to get b. So, we can also show that 3 is a factor of 12 by noting that $3 \times 4 = 12$.

Every positive whole number has 1 and itself as factors. If a whole number greater than one has *only* 1 and itself as factors, we call it a **prime number**. For instance, 5 is a prime number because its only factors are 1 and 5. The first several prime numbers are 2, 3, 5, 7, 11, and 13.

If a whole number greater than 1 is not prime—that is, if it has factors besides 1 and itself—then it is a **composite number.** For instance, 10 is a composite number because it has factors 2 and 5 in addition to 1 and 10. The first several composite numbers are 4, 6, 8, 9, 10, 12, 14, and 15.

A **prime factor** of a whole number is a factor that is also a prime number. For example, the prime factors of 12 are 2 and 3. The prime factors of 15 are 3 and 5.

A **common factor** of two (or more) whole numbers is a number that is a factor of both (or all) of them. For example, the factors of 12 are <u>1</u>, 2, <u>3</u>, 4, 6, and 12, while the factors of 15 are <u>1</u>, <u>3</u>, 5, and 15. The common factors (underlined) of 12 and 15 are 1 and 3.

The **greatest common factor** (**GCF**) of two (or more) whole numbers is the largest number that is a factor of both (or all) of them. For example, the factors of 15 are <u>1</u>, 3, <u>5</u>, and 15; the factors of 35 are <u>1</u>, <u>5</u>, 7, and 35. Therefore, the greatest common factor of 15 and 35 is 5.

Review Video: Factors
Visit mometrix.com/academy and enter code: 920086

Review Video: Prime Numbers and Factorization
Visit mometrix.com/academy and enter code: 760669

Multiples and Least Common Multiple

A whole number b is a **multiple** of a whole number a when a is a factor of b. This means that b is the product of a and another whole number. For example, the multiples of 7 are $0 \times 7 = 0, 1 \times 7 = 7, 2 \times 7 = 14, 3 \times 7 = 21, 4 \times 7 = 28, 5 \times 7 = 35, \ldots$. Dividing 0, 7, 14, 21, 28, and 35 by 7 results in the whole numbers 0, 1, 2, 3, 4, and 5, respectively, showing that 7 is a factor of these numbers.

The least common multiple (**LCM**) of two (or more) whole numbers is the smallest number that is a multiple of both (or all) of them. For example, the multiples of 3 are 3, 6, 9, 12, <u>15</u>, ...; the multiples of 5 are 5, 10, <u>15</u>, 20, ... The smallest number that appears in both lists is 15, so the least common multiple of 3 and 5 is 15.

Review Video: Multiples
Visit mometrix.com/academy and enter code: 626738

Review Video: Greatest Common Factor and Least Common Multiple
Visit mometrix.com/academy and enter code: 838699

Fractions

A **fraction** is a number that is expressed as one integer written above another integer, with a dividing line between them $\left(\frac{x}{y}\right)$. It represents the **quotient** of the two numbers "x divided by y." It can also be thought of as x out of y equal parts.

The top number of a fraction is called the **numerator**, and it represents the number of parts under consideration. The 1 in $\frac{1}{4}$ means that 1 part out of the whole is being considered in the calculation. The bottom number of a fraction is called the **denominator**, and it represents the total number of equal parts. The 4 in $\frac{1}{4}$ means that the whole consists of 4 equal parts. A fraction cannot have a denominator of zero; this is referred to as "*undefined*."

Fractions can be manipulated, without changing the value of the fraction, by multiplying or dividing (but not adding or subtracting) both the numerator and denominator by the same number. If you divide both numbers by a common factor, you are **reducing** or simplifying the fraction. Two fractions that have the same value but are expressed differently are known as **equivalent fractions**. For example, $\frac{2}{10}, \frac{3}{15}, \frac{4}{20}$, and $\frac{5}{25}$ are all equivalent fractions. They can also all be reduced or simplified to $\frac{1}{5}$.

When two fractions are manipulated so that they have the same denominator, this is known as finding a **common denominator**. The number chosen to be that common denominator should be the least common multiple of the two original denominators. Example: $\frac{3}{4}$ and $\frac{5}{6}$; the least common multiple of 4 and 6 is 12. Manipulating to achieve the common denominator: $\frac{3}{4} = \frac{9}{12}; \frac{5}{6} = \frac{10}{12}$.

Review Video: Overview of Fractions
Visit mometrix.com/academy and enter code: 262335

Proper Fractions and Mixed Numbers

A fraction whose denominator is greater than its numerator is known as a **proper fraction**, while a fraction whose numerator is greater than its denominator is known as an **improper fraction**. Proper fractions have values *less than one* and improper fractions have values *greater than one*.

A **mixed number** is a number that contains both an integer and a fraction. Any improper fraction can be rewritten as a mixed number. Example: $\frac{8}{3} = \frac{6}{3} + \frac{2}{3} = 2 + \frac{2}{3} = 2\frac{2}{3}$. Similarly, any mixed number can be rewritten as an improper fraction. Example: $1\frac{3}{5} = 1 + \frac{3}{5} = \frac{5}{5} + \frac{3}{5} = \frac{8}{5}$.

Review Video: Proper and Improper Fractions and Mixed Numbers
Visit mometrix.com/academy and enter code: 211077

Adding and Subtracting Fractions

If two fractions have a common denominator, they can be added or subtracted simply by adding or subtracting the two numerators and retaining the same denominator. If the two fractions do not already have the same denominator, one or both of them must be manipulated to achieve a common denominator before they can be added or subtracted. Example: $\frac{1}{2}+\frac{1}{4}=\frac{2}{4}+\frac{1}{4}=\frac{3}{4}$.

Review Video: Adding and Subtracting Fractions
Visit mometrix.com/academy and enter code: 378080

Multiplying Fractions

Two fractions can be multiplied by multiplying the two numerators to find the new numerator and the two denominators to find the new denominator. Example: $\frac{1}{3}\times\frac{2}{3}=\frac{1\times 2}{3\times 3}=\frac{2}{9}$.

Dividing Fractions

Two fractions can be divided by flipping the numerator and denominator of the second fraction and then proceeding as though it were a multiplication problem. Example: $\frac{2}{3}\div\frac{3}{4}=\frac{2}{3}\times\frac{4}{3}=\frac{8}{9}$.

Review Video: Multiplying and Dividing Fractions
Visit mometrix.com/academy and enter code: 473632

Multiplying a Mixed Number by a Whole Number or a Decimal

When multiplying a mixed number by something, it is usually best to convert it to an improper fraction first. Additionally, if the multiplicand is a decimal, it is most often simplest to convert it to a fraction. For instance, to multiply $4\frac{3}{8}$ by 3.5, begin by rewriting each quantity as a whole number plus a proper fraction. Remember, a mixed number is a fraction added to a whole number and a decimal is a representation of the sum of fractions, specifically tenths, hundredths, thousandths, and so on:

$$4\frac{3}{8}\times 3.5=\left(4+\frac{3}{8}\right)\times\left(3+\frac{1}{2}\right)$$

Next, the quantities being added need to be expressed with the same denominator. This is achieved by multiplying and dividing the whole number by the denominator of the fraction. Recall that a whole number is equivalent to that number divided by 1:

$$=\left(\frac{4}{1}\times\frac{8}{8}+\frac{3}{8}\right)\times\left(\frac{3}{1}\times\frac{2}{2}+\frac{1}{2}\right)$$

When multiplying fractions, remember to multiply the numerators and denominators separately:

$$=\left(\frac{4\times 8}{1\times 8}+\frac{3}{8}\right)\times\left(\frac{3\times 2}{1\times 2}+\frac{1}{2}\right)$$
$$=\left(\frac{32}{8}+\frac{3}{8}\right)\times\left(\frac{6}{2}+\frac{1}{2}\right)$$

Now that the fractions have the same denominators, they can be added:

$$=\frac{35}{8}\times\frac{7}{2}$$

Finally, perform the last multiplication and then simplify:

$$= \frac{35 \times 7}{8 \times 2} = \frac{245}{16} = \frac{240}{16} + \frac{5}{16} = 15\frac{5}{16}$$

COMPARING FRACTIONS

It is important to master the ability to compare and order fractions. This skill is relevant to many real-world scenarios. For example, carpenters often compare fractional construction nail lengths when preparing for a project, and bakers often compare fractional measurements to have the correct ratio of ingredients. There are three commonly used strategies when comparing fractions. These strategies are referred to as the common denominator approach, the decimal approach, and the cross-multiplication approach.

USING A COMMON DENOMINATOR TO COMPARE FRACTIONS

The fractions $\frac{2}{3}$ and $\frac{4}{7}$ have different denominators. $\frac{2}{3}$ has a denominator of 3, and $\frac{4}{7}$ has a denominator of 7. In order to precisely compare these two fractions, it is necessary to use a common denominator. A common denominator is a common multiple that is shared by both denominators. In this case, the denominators 3 and 7 share a multiple of 21. In general, it is most efficient to select the least common multiple for the two denominators.

Rewrite each fraction with the common denominator of 21. Then, calculate the new numerators as illustrated below.

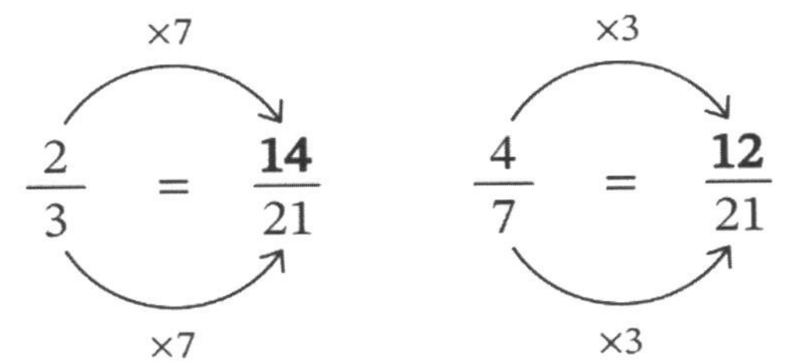

For $\frac{2}{3}$, multiply the numerator and denominator by 7. The result is $\frac{14}{21}$.

For $\frac{4}{7}$, multiply the numerator and denominator by 3. The result is $\frac{12}{21}$.

Now that both fractions have a denominator of 21, the fractions can accurately be compared by comparing the numerators. Since 14 is greater than 12, the fraction $\frac{14}{21}$ is greater than $\frac{12}{21}$. This means that $\frac{2}{3}$ is greater than $\frac{4}{7}$.

USING DECIMALS TO COMPARE FRACTIONS

Sometimes decimal values are easier to compare than fraction values. For example, $\frac{5}{8}$ is equivalent to 0.625 and $\frac{3}{5}$ is equivalent to 0.6. This means that the comparison of $\frac{5}{8}$ and $\frac{3}{5}$ can be determined by comparing the decimals 0.625 and 0.6. When both decimal values are extended to the thousandths place, they become 0.625 and 0.600, respectively. It becomes clear that 0.625 is greater than 0.600 because 625 thousandths is greater than 600 thousandths. In other words, $\frac{5}{8}$ is greater than $\frac{3}{5}$ because 0.625 is greater than 0.6.

Using Cross-Multiplication to Compare Fractions

Cross-multiplication is an efficient strategy for comparing fractions. This is a shortcut for the common denominator strategy. Start by writing each fraction next to one another. Multiply the numerator of the fraction on the left by the denominator of the fraction on the right. Write down the result next to the fraction on the left. Now multiply the numerator of the fraction on the right by the denominator of the fraction on the left. Write down the result next to the fraction on the right. Compare both products. The fraction with the larger result is the larger fraction.

Consider the fractions $\frac{4}{7}$ and $\frac{5}{9}$.

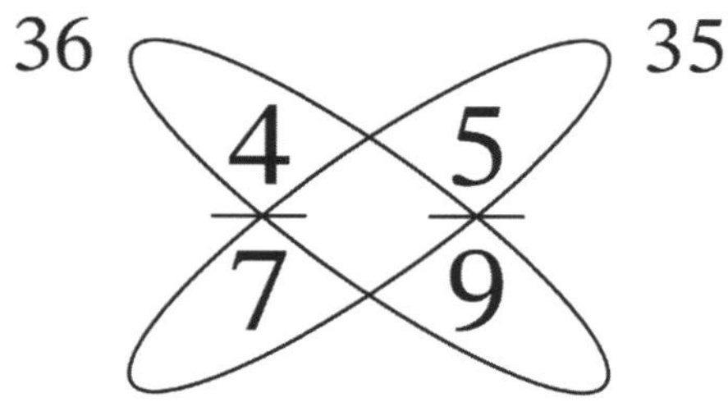

36 is greater than 35. Therefore, $\frac{4}{7}$ is greater than $\frac{5}{9}$.

Decimals

Decimals are one way to represent parts of a whole. Using the place value system, each digit to the right of a decimal point denotes the number of units of a corresponding *negative* power of ten. For example, consider the decimal 0.24. We can use a model to represent the decimal. Since a dime is worth one-tenth of a dollar and a penny is worth one-hundredth of a dollar, one possible model to represent this fraction is to have 2 dimes representing the 2 in the tenths place and 4 pennies representing the 4 in the hundredths place:

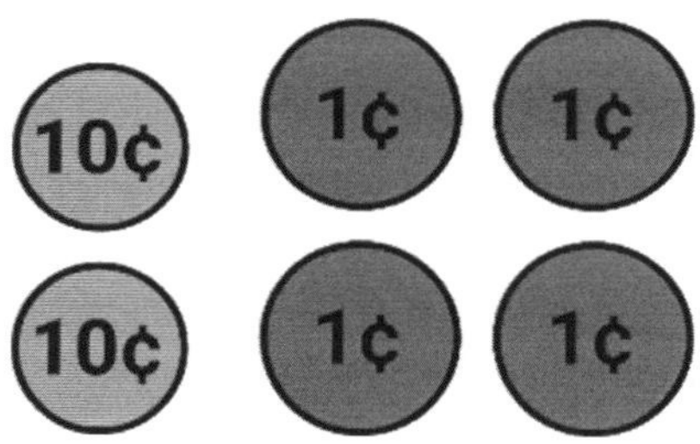

To write the decimal as a fraction, put the decimal in the numerator with 1 in the denominator. Multiply the numerator and denominator by tens until there are no more decimal places. Then simplify the fraction to lowest terms. For example, converting 0.24 to a fraction:

$$0.24 = \frac{0.24}{1} = \frac{0.24 \times 100}{1 \times 100} = \frac{24}{100} = \frac{6}{25}$$

Review Video: Decimals
Visit mometrix.com/academy and enter code: 837268

Operations with Decimals

Adding and Subtracting Decimals

When adding and subtracting decimals, the decimal points must always be aligned. Adding decimals is just like adding regular whole numbers. Example: $4.5 + 2.0 = 6.5$.

If the problem-solver does not properly align the decimal points, an incorrect answer of 4.7 may result. An easy way to add decimals is to align all of the decimal points in a vertical column visually. This will allow you to see exactly where the decimal should be placed in the final answer. Begin adding from right to left. Add each column in turn, making sure to carry the number to the left if a column adds up to more than 9. The same rules apply to the subtraction of decimals.

Review Video: Adding and Subtracting Decimals
Visit mometrix.com/academy and enter code: 381101

Multiplying Decimals

A simple multiplication problem has two components: a **multiplicand** and a **multiplier**. When multiplying decimals, work as though the numbers were whole rather than decimals. Once the final product is calculated, count the number of places to the right of the decimal in both the multiplicand and the multiplier. Then, count that number of places from the right of the product and place the decimal in that position.

For example, 12.3×2.56 has a total of three places to the right of the respective decimals. Multiply 123×256 to get 31,488. Now, beginning on the right, count three places to the left and insert the decimal. The final product will be 31.488.

Review Video: How to Multiply Decimals
Visit mometrix.com/academy and enter code: 731574

Dividing Decimals

Every division problem has a **divisor** and a **dividend**. The dividend is the number that is being divided. In the problem $14 \div 7$, 14 is the dividend and 7 is the divisor. In a division problem with decimals, the divisor must be converted into a whole number. Begin by moving the decimal in the divisor to the right until a whole number is created. Next, move the decimal in the dividend the same number of spaces to the right. For example, 4.9 into 24.5 would become 49 into 245. The decimal was moved one space to the right to create a whole number in the divisor, and then the same was done for the dividend. Once the whole numbers are created, the problem is carried out normally: $245 \div 49 = 5$.

Review Video: Dividing Decimals
Visit mometrix.com/academy and enter code: 560690

Review Video: Dividing Decimals by Whole Numbers
Visit mometrix.com/academy and enter code: 535669

Percentages

Percentages can be thought of as fractions that are based on a whole of 100; that is, one whole is equal to 100%. The word **percent** means "per hundred." Percentage problems are often presented in three main ways:

- Find what percentage of some number another number is.
  - Example: What percentage of 40 is 8?
- Find what number is some percentage of a given number.
  - Example: What number is 20% of 40?
- Find what number another number is a given percentage of.
  - Example: What number is 8 20% of?

There are three components in each of these cases: a **whole** (W), a **part** (P), and a **percentage** (%). These are related by the equation: $P = W \times \%$. This can easily be rearranged into other forms that may suit different questions better: $\% = \frac{P}{W}$ and $W = \frac{P}{\%}$. Percentage problems are often also word problems. As such, a large part of solving them is figuring out which quantities are what. For example, consider the following word problem:

In a school cafeteria, 7 students choose pizza, 9 choose hamburgers, and 4 choose tacos. What percentage of students choose tacos?

To find the whole, you must first add all of the parts: $7 + 9 + 4 = 20$. The percentage can then be found by dividing the part by the whole $\left(\% = \frac{P}{W}\right): \frac{4}{20} = \frac{20}{100} = 20\%$.

Review Video: Computation with Percentages
Visit mometrix.com/academy and enter code: 693099

Calculating Percent Change

Suppose a quantity has a particular value (the *old value*) and then we add something (the *change*) to it to get another value (the *new value*). We can describe this process by the simple equation $(\text{old value}) + \text{change} = (\text{new value})$. If we know the old and new values, we can rearrange this equation to find the change, getting $\text{change} = (\text{new value}) - (\text{old value})$. For instance, if a store's price for a box of computer paper goes from \$20 last week to \$25 this week, this is a change of $(\text{new value}) - (\text{old value}) = \$25 - \$20 = \$5$. Or, if the size of the freshman class at a college goes from 500 students one year to 440 students the next year, this is a change of $(\text{new value}) - (\text{old value}) = 440 - 500 = -60$ students. So, we see that change can be positive or negative.

Instead of the word *change*, we sometimes use the words *increase* or *decrease* to specify whether the value goes up or down, respectively. In the examples above, the price of computer paper increases by \$5 and the freshman class decreases by 60 students. Note that the decrease is 60 students and not -60 because the word *decrease* already means that the value goes down. So, *increase* is the same as positive change and *decrease* is the opposite or negative change.

If the changing quantity represents an amount (how much of something there is), we can also calculate the **percent change**. This is the change expressed as a percentage of the old amount. To calculate this, we divide the change by the old amount and express the quotient as a percent. That is, we use the formula $\text{percent change} = \frac{\text{change}}{\text{old value}}$, converting the resulting decimal answer to a percent. In the examples above, the price of a box of computer paper has a percent change of $\frac{\text{change in price}}{\text{old price}} = \frac{\$5}{\$20} = 0.25 = 25\%$, and the size of the freshman class at the college has a percent change of $\frac{\text{change in enrollment}}{\text{old enrollment}} = \frac{-60}{500} = -0.12 = -12\%$. We can also use the terms *percent increase* and *percent decrease*, saying that the price of computer paper increases by 25% and the size of the freshman class decreases by 12%. Note that the denominator is always the old amount, never the new amount.

Example: Your landlord raises your rent from $1,500 to $1,700 per month. To find the percent change in your rent (rounded to the nearest tenth of a percent), you calculate as follows.

$$\text{percent change in rent} = \frac{\text{change in rent}}{\text{old rent}} = \frac{(\text{new rent}) - (\text{old rent})}{\text{old rent}}$$
$$= \frac{\$1{,}700 - \$1{,}500}{\$1{,}500} = \frac{\$200}{\$1{,}500} = 0.1333\ldots \approx 13.3\%$$

Therefore, the percent change in your rent is approximately 13.3%.

Review Video: Percent Change
Visit mometrix.com/academy and enter code: 907890

Converting Between Percentages, Fractions, and Decimals

Converting decimals to percentages and percentages to decimals is as simple as moving the decimal point. To *convert from a decimal to a percentage*, move the decimal point **two places to the right**. To *convert from a percentage to a decimal*, move it **two places to the left**. It may be helpful to remember that the percentage number will always be larger than the equivalent decimal number. Example:

$$0.23 = 23\% \quad 5.34 = 534\% \quad 0.007 = 0.7\%$$
$$700\% = 7.00 \quad 86\% = 0.86 \quad 0.15\% = 0.0015$$

To convert a fraction to a decimal, simply divide the numerator by the denominator in the fraction. To convert a decimal to a fraction, put the decimal in the numerator with 1 in the denominator. Multiply the numerator and denominator by tens until there are no more decimal places. Then simplify the fraction to lowest terms. For example, converting 0.24 to a fraction:

$$0.24 = \frac{0.24}{1} = \frac{0.24 \times 100}{1 \times 100} = \frac{24}{100} = \frac{6}{25}$$

Fractions can be converted to a percentage by finding equivalent fractions with a denominator of 100. Example:

$$\frac{7}{10} = \frac{70}{100} = 70\% \quad \frac{1}{4} = \frac{25}{100} = 25\%$$

To convert a percentage to a fraction, divide the percentage number by 100 and reduce the fraction to its simplest possible terms. Example:

$$60\% = \frac{60}{100} = \frac{3}{5} \quad 96\% = \frac{96}{100} = \frac{24}{25}$$

Review Video: Converting Fractions to Percentages and Decimals
Visit mometrix.com/academy and enter code: 306233

Review Video: Converting Percentages to Decimals and Fractions
Visit mometrix.com/academy and enter code: 287297

Review Video: Converting Decimals to Fractions and Percentages
Visit mometrix.com/academy and enter code: 986765

Review Video: Converting Decimals, Improper Fractions, and Mixed Numbers
Visit mometrix.com/academy and enter code: 696924

Rational and Irrational Numbers

The term **rational** means that the number can be expressed as a ratio or fraction. That is, a number, r, is rational if and only if it can be represented by a fraction $\frac{a}{b}$ where a and b are integers and b does not equal 0. The set of rational numbers includes integers and decimals. If there is no finite way to represent a value with a fraction of integers, then the number is **irrational**. Common irrational numbers are π and the square roots of whole numbers that are not perfect squares (e.g., $\sqrt{5}$ or $\sqrt{21}$). The sum or product of an integer and an irrational number is always irrational (e.g., 3π or $7 + \sqrt{6}$).

Review Video: Rational and Irrational Numbers
Visit mometrix.com/academy and enter code: 280645

Review Video: Ordering Rational Numbers
Visit mometrix.com/academy and enter code: 419578

Review Video: Irrational Numbers on a Number Line
Visit mometrix.com/academy and enter code: 433866

Proportions and Ratios

Proportions

There is a **proportion** between two variable quantities if there is a constant relationship between their products or quotients, a relationship that does not change as the quantities themselves change.

Given variable quantities x and y, we say that they are **directly proportional** (or that y **varies directly with** x) if their quotient or *ratio* is constant—that is, if there is a constant k such that $\frac{y}{x} = k$ is always true. Another way of saying this is that y is a constant multiple of x, so that $y = kx$ is always true. We call the number k the **constant of proportionality**. For example, if you drive at a constant 50 miles per hour, then the distance, y, that you travel in miles is 50 times the number of hours, x, that you drive. In symbols, $y = 50x$ miles (or $\frac{y}{x} = 50$ mph). So, the distance you travel, y, is directly proportional to (or varies directly with) the time you travel, x, with constant of proportionality $k = 50$ mph.

The quantities x and y are **inversely proportional** (or y varies inversely with x) if their product is constant—that is, if there is a constant k such that $xy = k$ is always true. Another way of saying this is to say that y is a constant multiple of the reciprocal of x so that $y = \frac{k}{x}$ is always true. For instance, suppose you drive at speed (rate) y mph for x hours, going a total of 120 miles. Since rate × time = distance, we get $xy = 120$ miles (or $y = \frac{120}{x}$ miles per hour). Thus, your driving speed, y, is inversely proportional to (or varies inversely with) your drive time, x, with constant of proportionality $k = 120$ miles.

Review Video: Proportions
Visit mometrix.com/academy and enter code: 505355

Ratios

A **ratio** expresses the sizes of two quantities relative to each other. For instance, suppose we have 3 copies of sheet music to share among 6 singers. We can divide the singers into groups of 2 and give each group 1 copy of the music. Thus, there is 1 copy of the music for every 2 singers, and we say that the **ratio** of sheet music to singers is 1 to 2, which we write either as a fraction $\frac{1}{2}$ or using a colon 1 : 2. Of course, it is also true there are 3 copies for every 6 singers so that the ratio of sheet music to singers is also 3 to 6, which we write as $\frac{3}{6}$ or 3 : 6. So, the ratios $\frac{1}{2}$ and $\frac{3}{6}$ express the same relative quantities of music and singers. We say that these ratios are equal or **equivalent**, and we note that ratios are equal precisely when their fractions are equal (so, in this case, $\frac{1}{2} = \frac{3}{6}$ as fractions). We can also express the quantities in the other order and say that the ratio of singers to music is $\frac{2}{1}$ or 2 : 1 (or $\frac{6}{3}$ or 6 : 3).

Review Video: Ratios
Visit mometrix.com/academy and enter code: 996914

Constant of Proportionality

If variable quantities x and y are proportional and we know a pair of corresponding values for them, then we can find their constant of proportionality. If they are directly proportional, we use the formula $\frac{y}{x} = k$. If they are inversely proportional, we use the formula $xy = k$.

Example: The cost in dollars, y, of buying fence posts is directly proportional to the number, x, that you buy. If it costs $51 to buy 17 fence posts, what is the constant of proportionality? Because of direct proportionality, we know that $\frac{y}{x} = k$. Since this works for every pair of corresponding x- and y-values, it also works for $x = 17$ and $y = 51$. This gives us $\frac{51}{17} = k$, which simplifies to $k = 3$. Note also that this is the unit price, namely $3 per fence post.

WORK/UNIT RATE

Unit rate expresses a quantity of one thing in terms of one unit of another. For example, if you travel 30 miles every two hours, a unit rate expresses this comparison in terms of one hour: in one hour you travel 15 miles, so your unit rate is 15 miles per hour. Other examples are how much one ounce of food costs (price per ounce) or figuring out how much one egg costs out of the dozen (price per 1 egg, instead of price per 12 eggs). The denominator of a unit rate is always 1. Unit rates are used to compare different situations to solve problems. For example, to make sure you get the best deal when deciding which kind of soda to buy, you can find the unit rate of each. If soda #1 costs $1.50 for a 1-liter bottle, and soda #2 costs $2.75 for a 2-liter bottle, it would be a better deal to buy soda #2, because its unit rate is only $1.375 per liter, which is cheaper than soda #1. Unit rates can also help determine the length of time a given event will take. For example, if you can paint 2 rooms in 4.5 hours, you can determine how long it will take you to paint 5 rooms by solving for the unit rate per room and then multiplying that by 5.

Review Video: Rates and Unit Rates
Visit mometrix.com/academy and enter code: 185363

Chapter Quiz

Ready to see how well you retained what you just read? Scan the QR code to go directly to the chapter quiz interface for this study guide. If you're using a computer, simply visit the online resources page at **mometrix.com/resources719/pnat** and click the Chapter Quizzes link.

Language Ability

Parts of Speech

Nouns

A noun is a person, place, thing, or idea. The two main types of nouns are **common** and **proper** nouns. Nouns can also be categorized as abstract (i.e., general) or concrete (i.e., specific).

Common Nouns

Common nouns are generic names for people, places, and things. Common nouns are not usually capitalized.

Examples of common nouns:

People: boy, girl, worker, manager

Places: school, bank, library, home

Things: dog, cat, truck, car

Review Video: Nouns
Visit mometrix.com/academy and enter code: 344028

Proper Nouns

Proper nouns name specific people, places, or things. All proper nouns are capitalized.

Examples of proper nouns:

People: Abraham Lincoln, George Washington, Martin Luther King, Jr.

Places: Los Angeles, California; New York; Asia

Things: Statue of Liberty, Earth, Lincoln Memorial

Note: Some nouns can be either common or proper depending on their use. For example, when referring to the planet that we live on, *Earth* is a proper noun and is capitalized. When referring to the dirt, rocks, or land on our planet, *earth* is a common noun and is not capitalized.

General and Specific Nouns

General nouns are the names of conditions or ideas. **Specific nouns** name people, places, and things that are understood by using your senses.

General nouns:

Condition: beauty, strength

Idea: truth, peace

Specific nouns:

People: baby, friend, father

Places: town, park, city hall

Things: rainbow, cough, apple, silk, gasoline

Collective Nouns

Collective nouns are the names for a group of people, places, or things that may act as a whole. The following are examples of collective nouns: *class, company, dozen, group, herd, team,* and *public.* Collective nouns usually require an article, which denotes the noun as being a single unit. For instance, a choir is a group of singers. Even though there are many singers in a choir, the word choir is grammatically treated as a single unit. If we refer to the members of the group, and not the group itself, it is no longer a collective noun.

Incorrect: The *choir are* going to compete nationally this year.

Correct: The *choir is* going to compete nationally this year.

Incorrect: The *members* of the choir *is* competing nationally this year.

Correct: The *members* of the choir *are* competing nationally this year.

Pronouns

Pronouns are words that are used to stand in for nouns. A pronoun may be classified as personal, intensive, relative, interrogative, demonstrative, indefinite, and reciprocal.

Personal: *Nominative* is the case for nouns and pronouns that are the subject of a sentence. *Objective* is the case for nouns and pronouns that are an object in a sentence. *Possessive* is the case for nouns and pronouns that show possession or ownership.

Singular

	Nominative	Objective	Possessive
First Person	I	me	my, mine
Second Person	you	you	your, yours
Third Person	he, she, it	him, her, it	his, her, hers, its

Plural

	Nominative	Objective	Possessive
First Person	we	us	our, ours
Second Person	you	you	your, yours
Third Person	they	them	their, theirs

Intensive: I myself, you yourself, he himself, she herself, the (thing) itself, we ourselves, you yourselves, they themselves

Relative: which, who, whom, whose

Interrogative: what, which, who, whom, whose

Demonstrative: this, that, these, those

Indefinite: all, any, each, everyone, either/neither, one, some, several

Reciprocal: each other, one another

Review Video: Nouns and Pronouns
Visit mometrix.com/academy and enter code: 312073

VERBS

A verb is a word or group of words that indicates action or being. In other words, the verb shows something's action or state of being or the action that has been done to something. If you want to write a sentence, then you need a verb. Without a verb, you have no sentence.

TRANSITIVE AND INTRANSITIVE VERBS

A **transitive verb** is a verb whose action indicates a receiver. **Intransitive verbs** do not indicate a receiver of an action. In other words, the action of the verb does not point to an object.

Transitive: He drives a car. | She feeds the dog.

Intransitive: He runs every day. | She voted in the last election.

A dictionary will tell you whether a verb is transitive or intransitive. Some verbs can be transitive or intransitive.

ACTION VERBS AND LINKING VERBS

Action verbs show what the subject is doing. In other words, an action verb shows action. Unlike most types of words, a single action verb, in the right context, can be an entire sentence. **Linking verbs** link the subject of a sentence to a noun or pronoun, or they link a subject with an adjective. You always need a verb if you want a complete sentence. However, linking verbs on their own cannot be a complete sentence.

Common linking verbs include *appear, be, become, feel, grow, look, seem, smell, sound,* and *taste.* However, any verb that shows a condition and connects to a noun, pronoun, or adjective that describes the subject of a sentence is a linking verb.

Action: He sings. | Run! | Go! | I talk with him every day. | She reads.

Linking:

Incorrect: I am.

Correct: I am John. | The roses smell lovely. | I feel tired.

Note: Some verbs are followed by words that look like prepositions, but they are a part of the verb and a part of the verb's meaning. These are known as phrasal verbs, and examples include *call off*, *look up*, and *drop off*.

Review Video: Action Verbs and Linking Verbs
Visit mometrix.com/academy and enter code: 743142

Voice

Transitive verbs may be in active voice or passive voice. The difference between active voice and passive voice is whether the subject is acting or being acted upon. When the subject of the sentence is doing the action, the verb is in **active voice**. When the subject is being acted upon, the verb is in **passive voice**.

Active: Jon drew the picture. (The subject *Jon* is doing the action of *drawing a picture*.)

Passive: The picture is drawn by Jon. (The subject *picture* is receiving the action from Jon.)

Verb Tenses

Verb **tense** is a property of a verb that indicates when the action being described takes place (past, present, or future) and whether or not the action is completed (simple or perfect). Describing an action taking place in the present (*I talk*) requires a different verb tense than describing an action that took place in the past (*I talked*). Some verb tenses require an auxiliary (helping) verb. These helping verbs include *am, are, is* | *have, has, had* | *was, were, will* (or *shall*).

Present: I talk	Present perfect: I have talked
Past: I talked	Past perfect: I had talked
Future: I will talk	Future perfect: I will have talked

Present: The action is happening at the current time.

Example: He *walks* to the store every morning.

To show that something is happening right now, use the progressive present tense: I *am walking*.

Past: The action happened in the past.

Example: She *walked* to the store an hour ago.

Future: The action will happen later.

Example: I *will walk* to the store tomorrow.

Present perfect: The action started in the past and continues into the present or took place previously at an unspecified time.

Example: I *have walked* to the store three times today.

Past perfect: The action was completed at some point in the past. This tense is usually used to describe an action that was completed before some other reference time or event.

Example: I *had eaten* already before they arrived.

Future perfect: The action will be completed before some point in the future. This tense may be used to describe an action that has already begun or has yet to begin.

Example: The project *will have been completed* by the deadline.

Review Video: Present Perfect, Past Perfect, and Future Perfect Verb Tenses
Visit mometrix.com/academy and enter code: 269472

Conjugating Verbs

When you need to change the form of a verb, you are **conjugating** a verb. The key forms of a verb are present tense (sing/sings), past tense (sang), present participle (singing), and past participle (sung). By combining these forms with helping verbs, you can make almost any verb tense. The following table demonstrates some of the different ways to conjugate a verb:

Tense	First Person	Second Person	Third Person Singular	Third Person Plural
Simple Present	I sing	You sing	He, she, it sings	They sing
Simple Past	I sang	You sang	He, she, it sang	They sang
Simple Future	I will sing	You will sing	He, she, it will sing	They will sing
Present Progressive	I am singing	You are singing	He, she, it is singing	They are singing
Past Progressive	I was singing	You were singing	He, she, it was singing	They were singing
Present Perfect	I have sung	You have sung	He, she, it has sung	They have sung
Past Perfect	I had sung	You had sung	He, she, it had sung	They had sung

Mood

There are three **moods** in English: the indicative, the imperative, and the subjunctive.

The **indicative mood** is used for facts, opinions, and questions.

Fact: You can do this.

Opinion: I think that you can do this.

Question: Do you know that you can do this?

The **imperative** is used for orders or requests.

Order: You are going to do this!

Request: Will you do this for me?

The **subjunctive mood** is for wishes and statements that go against fact.

Wish: I wish that I were famous.

Statement against fact: If I were you, I would do this. (This goes against fact because I am not you. You have the chance to do this, and I do not have the chance.)

ADJECTIVES

An **adjective** is a word that is used to modify a noun or pronoun. An adjective answers a question: *Which one? What kind?* or *How many?* Usually, adjectives come before the words that they modify, but they may also come after a linking verb.

Which one? The *third* suit is my favorite.

What kind? This suit is *navy blue*.

How many? I am going to buy *four* pairs of socks to match the suit.

Review Video: Descriptive Text
Visit mometrix.com/academy and enter code: 174903

ARTICLES

Articles are adjectives that are used to distinguish nouns as definite or indefinite. *A*, *an*, and *the* are the only articles. **Definite** nouns are preceded by *the* and indicate a specific person, place, thing, or idea. **Indefinite** nouns are preceded by *a* or *an* and do not indicate a specific person, place, thing, or idea.

Note: *An* comes before words that start with a vowel sound. For example, "Are you going to get an **u**mbrella?"

Definite: I lost *the* bottle that belongs to me.

Indefinite: Does anyone have *a* bottle to share?

Review Video: Function of Articles in a Sentence
Visit mometrix.com/academy and enter code: 449383

COMPARISON WITH ADJECTIVES

Some adjectives are relative and other adjectives are absolute. Adjectives that are **relative** can show the comparison between things. **Absolute** adjectives can also show comparison, but they do so in a different way. Let's say that you are reading two books. You think that one book is perfect, and the other book is not exactly perfect. It is not possible for one book to be more perfect than the other. Either you think that the book is perfect, or you think that the book is imperfect. In this case, perfect and imperfect are absolute adjectives.

Relative adjectives will show the different **degrees** of something or someone to something else or someone else. The three degrees of adjectives include positive, comparative, and superlative.

The **positive** degree is the normal form of an adjective.

Example: This work is *difficult*. | She is *smart*.

The **comparative** degree compares one person or thing to another person or thing.

Example: This work is *more difficult* than your work. | She is *smarter* than me.

The **superlative** degree compares more than two people or things.

Example: This is the *most difficult* work of my life. | She is the *smartest* lady in school.

Review Video: Adjectives
Visit mometrix.com/academy and enter code: 470154

ADVERBS

An **adverb** is a word that is used to **modify** a verb, an adjective, or another adverb. Usually, adverbs answer one of these questions: *When? Where? How?* and *Why?* The negatives *not* and *never* are considered adverbs. Adverbs that modify adjectives or other adverbs **strengthen** or **weaken** the words that they modify.

Examples:

He walks *quickly* through the crowd.

The water flows *smoothly* on the rocks.

Note: Adverbs are usually indicated by the morpheme *-ly*, which has been added to the root word. For instance, *quick* can be made into an adverb by adding *-ly* to construct *quickly*. Some words that end in *-ly* do not follow this rule and can behave as other parts of speech. Examples of adjectives ending in *-ly* include: *early, friendly, holy, lonely, silly*, and *ugly*. To know if a word that ends in *-ly* is an adjective or adverb, check your dictionary. Also, while many adverbs end in *-ly*, you need to remember that not all adverbs end in *-ly*.

Examples:

He is *never* angry.

You are *too* irresponsible to travel alone.

Review Video: Adverbs
Visit mometrix.com/academy and enter code: 713951

Review Video: Adverbs that Modify Adjectives
Visit mometrix.com/academy and enter code: 122570

COMPARISON WITH ADVERBS

The rules for comparing adverbs are the same as the rules for adjectives.

The **positive** degree is the standard form of an adverb.

Example: He arrives *soon*. | She speaks *softly* to her friends.

The **comparative** degree compares one person or thing to another person or thing.

Example: He arrives *sooner* than Sarah. | She speaks *more softly* than him.

The **superlative** degree compares more than two people or things.

Example: He arrives *soonest* of the group. | She speaks the *most softly* of any of her friends.

Prepositions

A **preposition** is a word placed before a noun or pronoun that shows the relationship between that noun or pronoun and another word in the sentence.

Common prepositions:

about	before	during	on	under
after	beneath	for	over	until
against	between	from	past	up
among	beyond	in	through	with
around	by	of	to	within
at	down	off	toward	without

Examples:

The napkin is *in* the drawer.

The Earth rotates *around* the Sun.

The needle is *beneath* the haystack.

Can you find "me" *among* the words?

Review Video: Prepositions
Visit mometrix.com/academy and enter code: 946763

Conjunctions

Conjunctions join words, phrases, or clauses and they show the connection between the joined pieces. **Coordinating conjunctions** connect equal parts of sentences. **Correlative conjunctions** show the connection between pairs. **Subordinating conjunctions** join subordinate (i.e., dependent) clauses with independent clauses.

Coordinating Conjunctions

The **coordinating conjunctions** include: *and, but, yet, or, nor, for,* and *so*

Examples:

The rock was small, *but* it was heavy.

She drove in the night, *and* he drove in the day.

Correlative Conjunctions

The **correlative conjunctions** are: *either...or* | *neither...nor* | *not only...but also*

Examples:

Either you are coming *or* you are staying.

He *not only* ran three miles *but also* swam 200 yards.

Review Video: Coordinating and Correlative Conjunctions
Visit mometrix.com/academy and enter code: 390329

Review Video: Adverb Equal Comparisons
Visit mometrix.com/academy and enter code: 231291

Subordinating Conjunctions

Common **subordinating conjunctions** include:

after	since	whenever
although	so that	where
because	unless	wherever
before	until	whether
in order that	when	while

Examples:

I am hungry *because* I did not eat breakfast.

He went home *when* everyone left.

Review Video: Subordinating Conjunctions
Visit mometrix.com/academy and enter code: 958913

Interjections

Interjections are words of exclamation (i.e., audible expressions of great feeling) that are used alone or as a part of a sentence. Often, they are used at the beginning of a sentence for an introduction. Sometimes, they can be used in the middle of a sentence to show a change in thought or attitude.

Common Interjections: Hey! | Oh, | Ouch! | Please! | Wow!

Agreement and Sentence Structure

Subjects and Predicates

Subjects

The **subject** of a sentence names who or what the sentence is about. The subject may be directly stated in a sentence, or the subject may be the implied *you*. The **complete subject** includes the simple subject and all of its modifiers. To find the complete subject, ask *Who* or *What* and insert the verb to complete the question. The answer, including any modifiers (adjectives, prepositional phrases, etc.), is the complete subject. To find the **simple subject**, remove all of the modifiers in the complete subject. Being able to locate the subject of a sentence helps with many problems, such as those involving sentence fragments and subject-verb agreement.

Examples:

simple subject
The small, red car is the one that he wants for Christmas.
complete subject

simple subject
The young artist is coming over for dinner.
complete subject

Review Video: Subjects in English
Visit mometrix.com/academy and enter code: 444771

In **imperative** sentences, the verb's subject is understood (e.g., [You] Run to the store), but is not actually present in the sentence. Normally, the subject comes before the verb. However, the subject comes after the verb in sentences that begin with *There are* or *There was.*

Direct:

John knows the way to the park.	Who knows the way to the park?	John
The cookies need ten more minutes.	What needs ten minutes?	The cookies
By five o'clock, Bill will need to leave.	Who needs to leave?	Bill
There are five letters on the table for him.	What is on the table?	Five letters
There were coffee and doughnuts in the house.	What was in the house?	Coffee and doughnuts

Implied:

Go to the post office for me.	Who is going to the post office?	You
Come and sit with me, please?	Who needs to come and sit?	You

Predicates

In a sentence, you always have a predicate and a subject. The subject tells who or what the sentence is about, and the **predicate** explains or describes the subject. The predicate includes the verb or verb phrase and any direct or indirect objects of the verb, as well as any words or phrases modifying these.

Think about the sentence *He sings*. In this sentence, we have a subject (He) and a predicate (sings). This is all that is needed for a sentence to be complete. Most sentences contain more information, but if this is all the information that you are given, then you have a complete sentence.

Now, let's look at another sentence: *John and Jane sing on Tuesday nights at the dance hall.*

subject: John and Jane | predicate: sing on Tuesday nights at the dance hall.

John and Jane sing on Tuesday nights at the dance hall.

Review Video: Complete Predicate
Visit mometrix.com/academy and enter code: 293942

Subject-Verb Agreement

Verbs must **agree** with their subjects in number and in person. To agree in number, singular subjects need singular verbs and plural subjects need plural verbs. A **singular** noun refers to **one** person, place, or thing. A **plural** noun refers to **more than one** person, place, or thing. To agree in person, the correct verb form must be chosen to match the first, second, or third person subject. The present tense ending *-s* or *-es* is used on a verb if its subject is third person singular; otherwise, the verb's ending is not modified.

Review Video: Subject-Verb Agreement
Visit mometrix.com/academy and enter code: 479190

Number Agreement Examples:

Single Subject and Verb: Dan (singular subject) calls (singular verb) home.

Dan is one person. So, the singular verb *calls* is needed.

Plural Subject and Verb: Dan and Bob (plural subject) call (plural verb) home.

More than one person needs the plural verb *call.*

Person Agreement Examples:

First Person: I *am* walking.

Second Person: You *are* walking.

Third Person: He *is* walking.

Complications with Subject-Verb Agreement

Words Between Subject and Verb

Words that come between the simple subject and the verb have no bearing on subject-verb agreement.

Examples:

The joy (singular subject) of my life returns (singular verb) home tonight.

The phrase *of my life* does not influence the verb *returns.*

The question (singular subject) that still remains unanswered is (singular verb) "Who are you?"

Don't let the phrase "*that still remains…*" trouble you. The subject *question* goes with *is.*

Compound Subjects

A compound subject is formed when two or more nouns joined by *and, or,* or *nor* jointly act as the subject of the sentence.

Joined by And

When a compound subject is joined by *and,* it is treated as a plural subject and requires a plural verb.

Examples:

You and Jon (plural subject) are (plural verb) invited to come to my house.

The pencil and paper (plural subject) belong (plural verb) to me.

Joined by Or/Nor

For a compound subject joined by *or* or *nor,* the verb must agree in number with the part of the subject that is closest to the verb (italicized in the examples below).

Examples:

Today or tomorrow (subject) is (verb) the day.

Stan or Phil (subject) wants (verb) to read the book.

Neither the pen nor the book (subject) is (verb) on the desk.

Either the blanket or pillows (subject) arrive (verb) this afternoon.

INDEFINITE PRONOUNS AS SUBJECT

An indefinite pronoun is a pronoun that does not refer to a specific noun. Some indefinite pronouns function as only singular, some function as only plural, and some can function as either singular or plural depending on how they are used.

ALWAYS SINGULAR

Pronouns such as *each*, *either*, *everybody*, *anybody*, *somebody*, and *nobody* are always singular.

Examples:

singular subject — singular verb
Each of the runners has a different bib number.

singular verb — singular subject
Is either of you ready for the game?

Note: The words *each* and *either* can also be used as adjectives (e.g., *each* person is unique). When one of these adjectives modifies the subject of a sentence, it is always a singular subject.

singular subject — singular verb
Everybody grows a day older every day.

singular subject — singular verb
Anybody is welcome to bring a tent.

ALWAYS PLURAL

Pronouns such as *both*, *several*, and *many* are always plural.

Examples:

plural subject — plural verb
Both of the siblings were too tired to argue.

plural subject — plural verb
Many have tried, but none have succeeded.

DEPEND ON CONTEXT

Pronouns such as *some*, *any*, *all*, *none*, *more*, and *most* can be either singular or plural depending on what they are representing in the context of the sentence.

Examples:

singular subject — singular verb
All of my dog's food was still there in his bowl.

plural subject — plural verb
By the end of the night, all of my guests were already excited about coming to my next party.

OTHER CASES INVOLVING PLURAL OR IRREGULAR FORM

Some nouns are **singular in meaning but plural in form**: news, mathematics, physics, and economics.

The *news is* coming on now.

Mathematics is my favorite class.

Some nouns are plural in form and meaning, and have **no singular equivalent**: scissors and pants.

Do these *pants come* with a shirt?

The *scissors are* for my project.

Mathematical operations are **irregular** in their construction, but are normally considered to be **singular in meaning**.

One plus one is two.

Three times three is nine.

Note: Look to your **dictionary** for help when you aren't sure whether a noun with a plural form has a singular or plural meaning.

COMPLEMENTS

A complement is a noun, pronoun, or adjective that is used to give more information about the subject or object in the sentence.

DIRECT OBJECTS

A direct object is a noun or pronoun that tells who or what **receives** the action of the verb. A sentence will only include a direct object if the verb is a transitive verb. If the verb is an intransitive verb or a linking verb, there will be no direct object. When you are looking for a direct object, find the verb and ask *who* or *what*.

Examples:

I took *the blanket.*

Jane read *books.*

INDIRECT OBJECTS

An indirect object is a noun or pronoun that indicates what or whom the action had an **influence** on. If there is an indirect object in a sentence, then there will also be a direct object. When you are looking for the indirect object, find the verb and ask *to/for whom or what.*

Examples:

We taught [the old dog]indirect object [a new trick]direct object.

I gave [them]indirect object [a math lesson]direct object.

Review Video: Direct and Indirect Objects
Visit mometrix.com/academy and enter code: 817385

PREDICATE NOMINATIVES AND PREDICATE ADJECTIVES

As we looked at previously, verbs may be classified as either action verbs or linking verbs. A linking verb is so named because it links the subject to words in the predicate that describe or define the subject. These words are called predicate nominatives (if nouns or pronouns) or predicate adjectives (if adjectives).

Examples:

My [father]subject is a [lawyer]predicate nominative.

Your [mother]subject is [patient]predicate adjective.

PRONOUN USAGE

The **antecedent** is the noun that has been replaced by a pronoun. A pronoun and its antecedent **agree** when they have the same number (singular or plural) and gender (male, female, or neutral).

Examples:

Singular agreement: [John]antecedent came into town, and [he]pronoun played for us.

Plural agreement: [John and Rick]antecedent came into town, and [they]pronoun played for us.

To determine which is the correct pronoun to use in a compound subject or object, try each pronoun **alone** in place of the compound in the sentence. Your knowledge of pronouns will tell you which one is correct.

Example:

Bob and (I, me) will be going.

Test: (1) *I will be going* or (2) *Me will be going*. The second choice cannot be correct because *me* cannot be used as the subject of a sentence. Instead, *me* is used as an object.

Answer: Bob and I will be going.

When a pronoun is used with a noun immediately following (as in "we boys"), try the sentence **without the added noun**.

Example:

(We/Us) boys played football last year.

Test: (1) *We played football last ye*ar or (2) *Us played football last year*. Again, the second choice cannot be correct because *us* cannot be used as a subject of a sentence. Instead, *us* is used as an object.

Answer: We boys played football last year.

Review Video: Pronoun Usage
Visit mometrix.com/academy and enter code: 666500

Review Video: Pronoun-Antecedent Agreement
Visit mometrix.com/academy and enter code: 919704

A pronoun should point clearly to the **antecedent**. Here is how a pronoun reference can be unhelpful if it is puzzling or not directly stated.

Unhelpful: Ron and Jim (antecedent) went to the store, and he (pronoun) bought soda.

Who bought soda? Ron or Jim?

Helpful: Jim (antecedent) went to the store, and he (pronoun) bought soda.

The sentence is clear. Jim bought the soda.

Some pronouns change their form by their placement in a sentence. A pronoun that is a **subject** in a sentence comes in the **subjective case**. Pronouns that serve as **objects** appear in the **objective case**. Finally, the pronouns that are used as **possessives** appear in the **possessive case**.

Examples:

Subjective case: *He* is coming to the show.

The pronoun *He* is the subject of the sentence.

Objective case: Josh drove *him* to the airport.

The pronoun *him* is the object of the sentence.

Possessive case: The flowers are *mine*.

The pronoun *mine* shows ownership of the flowers.

The word *who* is a subjective-case pronoun that can be used as a **subject**. The word *whom* is an objective-case pronoun that can be used as an **object**. The words *who* and *whom* are common in subordinate clauses or in questions.

Examples:

He knows who (subject) wants (verb) to come.

He knows the man whom (object) we want (verb) at the party.

Clauses

A clause is a group of words that contains both a subject and a predicate (verb). There are two types of clauses: independent and dependent. An **independent clause** contains a complete thought, while a **dependent (or subordinate) clause** does not. A dependent clause includes a subject and a verb, and may also contain objects or complements, but it cannot stand as a complete thought without being joined to an independent clause. Dependent clauses function within sentences as adjectives, adverbs, or nouns.

Example:

I am running (independent clause) because I want to stay in shape. (dependent clause)

The clause *I am running* is an independent clause: it has a subject and a verb, and it gives a complete thought. The clause *because I want to stay in shape* is a dependent clause: it has a subject and a verb, but it does not express a complete thought. It adds detail to the independent clause to which it is attached.

Review Video: Clauses
Visit mometrix.com/academy and enter code: 940170

Review Video: Independent and Dependent Clauses
Visit mometrix.com/academy and enter code: 556903

Types of Dependent Clauses

Adjective Clauses

An **adjective clause** is a dependent clause that modifies a noun or a pronoun. Adjective clauses begin with a relative pronoun (*who, whose, whom, which,* and *that*) or a relative adverb (*where, when,* and *why*).

Also, adjective clauses usually come immediately after the noun that the clause needs to explain or rename. This is done to ensure that it is clear which noun or pronoun the clause is modifying.

Examples:

I learned the reason (independent clause) why I won the award. (adjective clause)

This is the place (independent clause) where I started my first job. (adjective clause)

An adjective clause can be an essential or nonessential clause. An essential clause is very important to the sentence. **Essential clauses** explain or define a person or thing. **Nonessential clauses** give more information about a person or thing but are not necessary to define them. Nonessential clauses are set off with commas while essential clauses are not.

Examples:

A person who works hard at first (essential clause) can often rest later in life.

Neil Armstrong, who walked on the moon, (nonessential clause) is my hero.

Review Video: Adjective Clauses and Phrases
Visit mometrix.com/academy and enter code: 520888

Adverb Clauses

An **adverb clause** is a dependent clause that modifies a verb, adjective, or adverb. In sentences with multiple dependent clauses, adverb clauses are usually placed immediately before or after the independent clause. An adverb clause is introduced with words such as *after, although, as, before, because, if, since, so, unless, when, where*, and *while*.

Examples:

When you walked outside, (adverb clause) I called the manager.

I will go with you unless you want to stay. (adverb clause)

Noun Clauses

A **noun clause** is a dependent clause that can be used as a subject, object, or complement. Noun clauses begin with words such as *how, that, what, whether, which, who,* and *why*. These words can also come with an adjective clause. Unless the noun clause is being used as the subject of the sentence, it should come after the verb of the independent clause.

Examples:

> noun clause
> The real mystery is how you avoided serious injury.

> noun clause
> What you learn from each other depends on your honesty with others.

Subordination

When two related ideas are not of equal importance, the ideal way to combine them is to make the more important idea an independent clause and the less important idea a dependent or subordinate clause. This is called **subordination**.

Example:

> **Separate ideas**: The team had a perfect regular season. The team lost the championship.
>
> **Subordinated**: Despite having a perfect regular season, *the team lost the championship*.

Phrases

A phrase is a group of words that functions as a single part of speech, usually a noun, adjective, or adverb. A **phrase** is not a complete thought and does not contain a subject and predicate, but it adds detail or explanation to a sentence, or renames something within the sentence.

Prepositional Phrases

One of the most common types of phrases is the prepositional phrase. A **prepositional phrase** begins with a preposition and ends with a noun or pronoun that is the object of the preposition. Normally, the prepositional phrase functions as an **adjective** or an **adverb** within the sentence.

Examples:

> prepositional phrase
> The picnic is on the blanket.

> prepositional phrase
> I am sick with a fever today.

> prepositional phrase
> Among the many flowers, John found a four-leaf clover.

Verbal Phrases

A **verbal** is a word or phrase that is formed from a verb but does not function as a verb. Depending on its particular form, it may be used as a noun, adjective, or adverb. A verbal does **not** replace a verb in a sentence.

Examples:

> verb
> Correct: Walk a mile daily.
>
> This is a complete sentence with the implied subject *you*.

verbal
Incorrect: To walk a mile.

This is not a sentence since there is no functional verb.

There are three types of verbal: **participles**, **gerunds**, and **infinitives**. Each type of verbal has a corresponding **phrase** that consists of the verbal itself along with any complements or modifiers.

Participles

A **participle** is a type of verbal that always functions as an adjective. The present participle always ends with *-ing*. Past participles end with *-d, -ed, -n,* or *-t*. Participles are combined with helping verbs to form certain verb tenses, but a participle by itself cannot function as a verb.

Examples: dance (verb) | dancing (present participle) | danced (past participle)

Participial phrases most often come right before or right after the noun or pronoun that they modify.

Examples:

Shipwrecked on an island (participial phrase), the boys started to fish for food.

Having been seated for five hours (participial phrase), we got out of the car to stretch our legs.

Praised for their work (participial phrase), the group accepted the first-place trophy.

Gerunds

A **gerund** is a type of verbal that always functions as a **noun**. Like present participles, gerunds always end with *-ing*, but they can be easily distinguished from participles by the part of speech they represent (participles always function as adjectives). Since a gerund or gerund phrase always functions as a noun, it can be used as the subject of a sentence, the predicate nominative, or the object of a verb or preposition.

Examples:

We want to be known for teaching (gerund) the poor (teaching the poor: object of preposition).

Coaching (gerund) this team (Coaching this team: subject) is the best job of my life.

We like practicing (gerund) our songs (practicing our songs: object of verb) in the basement.

INFINITIVES

An **infinitive** is a type of verbal that can function as a noun, an adjective, or an adverb. An infinitive is made of the word *to* and the basic form of the verb. As with all other types of verbal phrases, an infinitive phrase includes the verbal itself and all of its complements or modifiers.

Examples:

infinitive
To join the team is my goal in life.
noun

infinitive
The animals have enough food to eat for the night.
adjective

infinitive
People lift weights to exercise their muscles.
adverb

Review Video: Verbals
Visit mometrix.com/academy and enter code: 915480

APPOSITIVE PHRASES

An **appositive** is a word or phrase that is used to explain or rename nouns or pronouns. Noun phrases, gerund phrases, and infinitive phrases can all be used as appositives.

Examples:

appositive
Terriers, hunters at heart, have been dressed up to look like lap dogs.

The noun phrase *hunters at heart* renames the noun *terriers*.

appositive
His plan, to save and invest his money, was proven as a safe approach.

The infinitive phrase explains what the plan is.

Appositive phrases can be **essential** or **nonessential**. An appositive phrase is essential if the person, place, or thing being described or renamed is too general for its meaning to be understood without the appositive.

Examples:

essential
Two of America's Founding Fathers, George Washington and Thomas Jefferson, served as presidents.

nonessential
George Washington and Thomas Jefferson, two Founding Fathers, served as presidents.

ABSOLUTE PHRASES

An absolute phrase is a phrase that consists of **a noun followed by a participle**. An absolute phrase provides **context** to what is being described in the sentence, but it does not modify or explain any particular word; it is essentially independent.

Examples:

noun participle
The alarm ringing, he pushed the snooze button.
absolute phrase

noun participle
The music paused, she continued to dance through the crowd.
absolute phrase

PARALLELISM

When multiple items or ideas are presented in a sentence in series, such as in a list, the items or ideas must be stated in grammatically equivalent ways. For example, if two ideas are listed in parallel and the first is stated in gerund form, the second cannot be stated in infinitive form. (e.g., *I enjoy reading and to study.* [incorrect]) An infinitive and a gerund are not grammatically equivalent. Instead, you should write *I enjoy reading and studying* OR *I like to read and to study*. In lists of more than two, all items must be parallel.

Example:

> **Incorrect**: He stopped at the office, grocery store, and the pharmacy before heading home.
>
> The first and third items in the list of places include the article *the*, so the second item needs it as well.
>
> **Correct**: He stopped at the office, *the* grocery store, and the pharmacy before heading home.

Example:

> **Incorrect**: While vacationing in Europe, she went biking, skiing, and climbed mountains.
>
> The first and second items in the list are gerunds, so the third item must be as well.
>
> **Correct**: While vacationing in Europe, she went biking, skiing, and *mountain climbing*.

Review Video: Parallel Sentence Construction
Visit mometrix.com/academy and enter code: 831988

SENTENCE PURPOSE

There are four types of sentences: declarative, imperative, interrogative, and exclamatory.

A **declarative** sentence states a fact and ends with a period.

> *The football game starts at seven o'clock.*

An **imperative** sentence tells someone to do something and generally ends with a period. An urgent command might end with an exclamation point instead.

> *Don't forget to buy your ticket.*

An **interrogative** sentence asks a question and ends with a question mark.

> *Are you going to the game on Friday?*

An **exclamatory** sentence shows strong emotion and ends with an exclamation point.

> *I can't believe we won the game!*

Sentence Structure

Sentences are classified by structure based on the type and number of clauses present. The four classifications of sentence structure are the following:

Simple: A simple sentence has one independent clause with no dependent clauses. A simple sentence may have **compound elements** (i.e., compound subject or verb).

Examples:

single subject	single verb	
Judy	watered	the lawn.

compound subject	single verb	
Judy and Alan	watered	the lawn.

single subject	compound verb		compound verb	
Judy	watered	the lawn and	pulled	weeds.

compound subject	compound verb		compound verb	
Judy and Alan	watered	the lawn and	pulled	weeds.

Compound: A compound sentence has two or more independent clauses with no dependent clauses. Usually, the independent clauses are joined with a comma and a coordinating conjunction or with a semicolon.

Examples:

independent clause		independent clause
The time has come,	and	we are ready.

independent clause	independent clause
I woke up at dawn;	the sun was just coming up.

Complex: A complex sentence has one independent clause and at least one dependent clause. Punctuation depends on whether the dependent (subordinate) clause comes before or after the independent (or main) clause. If the subordinate clause comes first, it needs to be set apart with a comma.

Examples:

Although he had the flu, (dependent clause) Harry went to work. (independent clause)

Marcia got married (independent clause) after she finished college. (dependent clause)

Compound-Complex: A compound-complex sentence has at least two independent clauses and at least one dependent clause.

Examples:

John is my friend (independent clause) who went to India, (dependent clause) and he brought back souvenirs. (independent clause)

You may not realize this, (independent clause) but we heard the music (independent clause) that you played last night. (dependent clause)

Review Video: Sentence Structure
Visit mometrix.com/academy and enter code: 700478

Sentence variety is important to consider when writing an essay or speech. A variety of sentence lengths and types creates rhythm, makes a passage more engaging, and gives writers an opportunity to demonstrate their writing style. Writing that uses the same length or type of sentence without variation can be boring or difficult to read. To evaluate a passage for effective sentence variety, it is helpful to note whether the passage contains diverse sentence structures and lengths. It is also important to pay attention to the way each sentence starts and avoid beginning with the same words or phrases.

Sentence Fragments

Recall that a group of words must contain at least one **independent clause** in order to be considered a sentence. If it doesn't contain even one independent clause, it is called a **sentence fragment**.

The appropriate process for **repairing** a sentence fragment depends on what type of fragment it is. If the fragment is a dependent clause, it can sometimes be as simple as removing a subordinating word (e.g., when, because, if) from the beginning of the fragment. Alternatively, a dependent clause can be incorporated into a closely related neighboring sentence. If the fragment is missing some required part, like a subject or a verb, the fix might be as simple as adding the missing part.

Examples:

Fragment: Because he wanted to sail the Mediterranean.

Removed subordinating word: He wanted to sail the Mediterranean.

Combined with another sentence: Because he wanted to sail the Mediterranean, he booked a Greek island cruise.

RUN-ON SENTENCES

Run-on sentences consist of multiple independent clauses that have not been joined together properly. Run-on sentences can be corrected in several different ways:

Join clauses properly: This can be done with a comma and coordinating conjunction, with a semicolon, or with a colon or dash if the second clause is explaining something in the first.

Example:

Incorrect: I went on the trip, we visited lots of castles.

Corrected: I went on the trip, and we visited lots of castles.

Split into separate sentences: This correction is most effective when the independent clauses are very long or when they are not closely related.

Example:

Incorrect: The drive to New York takes ten hours, my uncle lives in Boston.

Corrected: The drive to New York takes ten hours. My uncle lives in Boston.

Make one clause dependent: This is the easiest way to make the sentence correct and more interesting at the same time. It's often as simple as adding a subordinating word between the two clauses or before the first clause.

Example:

Incorrect: I finally made it to the store and I bought some eggs.

Corrected: When I finally made it to the store, I bought some eggs.

Reduce to one clause with a compound verb: If both clauses have the same subject, remove the subject from the second clause, and you now have just one clause with a compound verb.

Example:

Incorrect: The drive to New York takes ten hours, it makes me very tired.

Corrected: The drive to New York takes ten hours and makes me very tired.

Note: While these are the simplest ways to correct a run-on sentence, often the best way is to completely reorganize the thoughts in the sentence and rewrite it.

Review Video: Fragments and Run-on Sentences
Visit mometrix.com/academy and enter code: 541989

Dangling and Misplaced Modifiers

Dangling Modifiers

A dangling modifier is a dependent clause or verbal phrase that does not have a clear logical connection to a word in the sentence.

Example:

Incorrect: Reading each magazine article [dangling modifier], the stories caught my attention.

The word *stories* cannot be modified by *Reading each magazine article*. People can read, but stories cannot read. Therefore, the subject of the sentence must be a person.

Corrected: Reading each magazine article [gerund phrase], I was entertained by the stories.

Example:

Incorrect: Ever since childhood [dangling modifier], my grandparents have visited me for Christmas.

The speaker in this sentence can't have been visited by her grandparents when *they* were children, since she wouldn't have been born yet. Either the modifier should be clarified or the sentence should be rearranged to specify whose childhood is being referenced.

Clarified: Ever since I was a child [dependent clause], my grandparents have visited for Christmas.

Rearranged: Ever since childhood [adverb phrase], I have enjoyed my grandparents visiting for Christmas.

Misplaced Modifiers

Because modifiers are grammatically versatile, they can be put in many different places within the structure of a sentence. The danger of this versatility is that a modifier can accidentally be placed where it is modifying the wrong word or where it is not clear which word it is modifying.

Example:

Incorrect: She read the book to a crowd that was filled with beautiful pictures [modifier].

The book was filled with beautiful pictures, not the crowd.

Corrected: She read the book that was filled with beautiful pictures (modifier) to a crowd.

Example:

Ambiguous: Derek saw a bus nearly hit a man on his way to work. (modifier: on his way to work)

Was Derek on his way to work or was the other man?

Derek: On his way to work, (modifier) Derek saw a bus nearly hit a man.

The other man: Derek saw a bus nearly hit a man who was on his way to work. (modifier: who was on his way to work)

Split Infinitives

A split infinitive occurs when a modifying word comes between the word *to* and the verb that pairs with *to*.

Example: To *clearly* explain vs. *To explain* clearly | To *softly* sing vs. *To sing* softly

Though considered improper by some, split infinitives may provide better clarity and simplicity in some cases than the alternatives. As such, avoiding them should not be considered a universal rule.

Double Negatives

Standard English allows **two negatives** only when a **positive** meaning is intended. (e.g., The team was *not displeased* with their performance.) Double negatives to emphasize negation are not used in standard English.

Negative modifiers (e.g., never, no, and not) should not be paired with other negative modifiers or negative words (e.g., none, nobody, nothing, or neither). The modifiers *hardly, barely*, and *scarcely* are also considered negatives in standard English, so they should not be used with other negatives.

Punctuation

End Punctuation

Periods

Use a period to end all sentences except direct questions and exclamations. Periods are also used for abbreviations.

Examples: 3 p.m. | 2 a.m. | Mr. Jones | Mrs. Stevens | Dr. Smith | Bill, Jr. | Pennsylvania Ave.

Note: An abbreviation is a shortened form of a word or phrase.

Question Marks

Question marks should be used following a **direct question**. A polite request can be followed by a period instead of a question mark.

Direct Question: What is for lunch today? | How are you? | Why is that the answer?

Polite Requests: Can you please send me the item tomorrow. | Will you please walk with me on the track.

Review Video: Question Marks
Visit mometrix.com/academy and enter code: 118471

Exclamation Marks

Exclamation marks are used after a word group or sentence that shows much feeling or has special importance. Exclamation marks should not be overused. They are saved for proper **exclamatory interjections**.

Example: We're going to the finals! | You have a beautiful car! | "That's crazy!" she yelled.

Review Video: Exclamation Points
Visit mometrix.com/academy and enter code: 199367

Commas

The comma is a punctuation mark that can help you understand connections in a sentence. Not every sentence needs a comma. However, if a sentence needs a comma, you need to put it in the right place. A comma in the wrong place (or an absent comma) will make a sentence's meaning unclear.

These are some of the rules for commas:

Use Case	Example
Before a **coordinating conjunction** joining independent clauses	Bob caught three fish, and I caught two fish.
After an **introductory phrase**	After the final out, we went to a restaurant to celebrate.
After an **adverbial clause**	Studying the stars, I was awed by the beauty of the sky.
Between **items in a series**	I will bring the turkey, the pie, and the coffee.
For **interjections**	Wow, you know how to play this game.
After ***yes*** **and** ***no*** **responses**	No, I cannot come tomorrow.
Separate **nonessential modifiers**	John Frank, who coaches the team, was promoted today.
Separate **nonessential appositives**	Thomas Edison, an American inventor, was born in Ohio.
Separate **nouns of direct address**	You, John, are my only hope in this moment.
Separate **interrogative tags**	This is the last time, correct?
Separate **contrasts**	You are my friend, not my enemy.
Writing **dates**	July 4, 1776, is an important date to remember.
Writing **addresses**	He is meeting me at 456 Delaware Avenue, Washington, D.C., tomorrow morning.
Writing **geographical names**	Paris, France, is my favorite city.
Writing **titles**	John Smith, PhD, will be visiting your class today.
Separate **expressions like** ***he said***	"You can start," she said, "with an apology."

A comma is also used **between coordinate adjectives** not joined with *and*. However, not all adjectives are coordinate (i.e., equal or parallel). To determine if your adjectives are coordinate, try connecting them with *and* or reversing their order. If it still sounds right, they are coordinate.

Incorrect: The kind, brown dog followed me home.

Correct: The kind, loyal dog followed me home.

Review Video: When to Use a Comma
Visit mometrix.com/academy and enter code: 786797

SEMICOLONS

The semicolon is used to join closely related independent clauses without the need for a coordinating conjunction. Semicolons are also used in place of commas to separate list elements that have internal commas. Some rules for semicolons include:

Use Case	Example
Between closely connected independent clauses **not connected with a coordinating conjunction**	You are right; we should go with your plan.
Between independent clauses **linked with a transitional word**	I think that we can agree on this; however, I am not sure about my friends.
Between items in a **series that has internal punctuation**	I have visited New York, New York; Augusta, Maine; and Baltimore, Maryland.

Review Video: How to Use Semicolons
Visit mometrix.com/academy and enter code: 370605

COLONS

The colon is used to call attention to the words that follow it. When used in a sentence, a colon should only come at the **end** of a **complete sentence**. The rules for colons are as follows:

Use Case	Example
After an independent clause to **make a list**	I want to learn many languages: Spanish, German, and Italian.
For **explanations**	There is one thing that stands out on your resume: responsibility.
To give a **quote**	He started with an idea: "We are able to do more than we imagine."
After the **greeting in a formal letter**	To Whom It May Concern:
Show **hours and minutes**	It is 3:14 p.m.
Separate a **title and subtitle**	The essay is titled "America: A Short Introduction to a Modern Country."

Review Video: Using Colons
Visit mometrix.com/academy and enter code: 868673

PARENTHESES

Parentheses are used for additional information. Also, they can be used to put labels for letters or numbers in a series. Parentheses should not be used very often. If they are overused, parentheses can be a distraction instead of a help.

Examples:

Extra Information: The rattlesnake (see Image 2) is a dangerous snake of North and South America.

Series: Include in the email (1) your name, (2) your address, and (3) your question for the author.

Review Video: Parentheses
Visit mometrix.com/academy and enter code: 947743

QUOTATION MARKS

Use quotation marks to close off **direct quotations** of a person's spoken or written words. Do not use quotation marks around indirect quotations. An indirect quotation gives someone's message without using the person's exact words. Use **single quotation marks** to close off a quotation inside a quotation.

Direct Quote: Nancy said, "I am waiting for Henry to arrive."

Indirect Quote: Henry said that he is going to be late to the meeting.

Quote inside a Quote: The teacher asked, "Has everyone read 'The Gift of the Magi'?"

Quotation marks should be used around the titles of **short works**: newspaper and magazine articles, poems, short stories, songs, television episodes, radio programs, and subdivisions of books or websites.

Examples:

"Rip Van Winkle" (short story by Washington Irving)

"O Captain! My Captain!" (poem by Walt Whitman)

Although it is not standard usage, quotation marks are sometimes used to highlight **irony** or the use of words to mean something other than their dictionary definition. This type of usage should be employed sparingly, if at all.

Examples:

The boss warned Frank that he was walking on "thin ice."	Frank is not walking on real ice. Instead, he is being warned to avoid mistakes.
The teacher thanked the young man for his "honesty."	The quotation marks around *honesty* show that the teacher does not believe the young man's explanation.

Review Video: Quotation Marks
Visit mometrix.com/academy and enter code: 884918

Periods and commas are put **inside** quotation marks. Colons and semicolons are put **outside** the quotation marks. Question marks and exclamation points are placed inside quotation marks when they are part of a quote. When the question or exclamation mark goes with the whole sentence, the mark is left outside of the quotation marks.

Examples:

Period and comma	We read "The Gift of the Magi," "The Skylight Room," and "The Cactus."
Semicolon	They watched "The Nutcracker"; then, they went home.
Exclamation mark that is a part of a quote	The crowd cheered, "Victory!"
Question mark that goes with the whole sentence	Is your favorite short story "The Tell-Tale Heart"?

APOSTROPHES

An apostrophe is used to show **possession** or the **deletion of letters in contractions**. An apostrophe is not needed with the possessive pronouns *his, hers, its, ours, theirs, whose*, and *yours*.

Singular Nouns: David's car | a book's theme | my brother's board game

Plural Nouns that end with -*s*: the scissors' handle | boys' basketball

Plural Nouns that end without -*s*: Men's department | the people's adventure

Review Video: When to Use an Apostrophe
Visit mometrix.com/academy and enter code: 213068

Review Video: Punctuation Errors in Possessive Pronouns
Visit mometrix.com/academy and enter code: 221438

HYPHENS

Hyphens are used to **separate compound words**. Use hyphens in the following cases:

Use Case	Example
Compound numbers from 21 to 99 when written out in words	This team needs twenty-five points to win the game.
Written-out fractions that are used as adjectives	The recipe says that we need a three-fourths cup of butter.
Compound adjectives that come before a noun	The well-fed dog took a nap.
Unusual compound words that would be hard to read or easily confused with other words	This is the best anti-itch cream on the market.

Note: This is not a complete set of the rules for hyphens. A dictionary is the best tool for knowing if a compound word needs a hyphen.

Review Video: Hyphens
Visit mometrix.com/academy and enter code: 981632

DASHES

Dashes are used to show a **break** or a **change in thought** in a sentence or to act as parentheses in a sentence. When typing, use two hyphens to make a dash. Do not put a space before or after the dash. The following are the functions of dashes:

Use Case	Example
Set off parenthetical statements or an **appositive with internal punctuation**	The three trees—oak, pine, and magnolia—are coming on a truck tomorrow.
Show a **break or change in tone or thought**	The first question—how silly of me—does not have a correct answer.

ELLIPSIS MARKS

The ellipsis mark has **three** periods (…) to show when **words have been removed** from a quotation. If a **full sentence or more** is removed from a quoted passage, you need to use **four** periods to show the removed text and the end punctuation mark. The ellipsis mark should not be used at the beginning of a quotation. The ellipsis mark should also not be used at the end of a quotation unless some words have been deleted from the end of the final quoted sentence.

Example:

> "Then he picked up the groceries…paid for them…later he went home."

BRACKETS

There are two main reasons to use brackets:

Use Case	Example
Placing **parentheses inside of parentheses**	The hero of this story, Paul Revere (a silversmith and industrialist [see Ch. 4]), rode through towns of Massachusetts to warn of advancing British troops.
Adding **clarification or detail to a quotation** that is not part of the quotation	The father explained, "My children are planning to attend my alma mater [State University]."

Review Video: Brackets
Visit mometrix.com/academy and enter code: 727546

Common Usage Mistakes

Commonly Confused Words

Which, That, and Who

The words *which, that,* and *who* can act as **relative pronouns** to help clarify or describe a noun.

Which is used for things only.

Example: Andrew's car, *which is old and rusty,* broke down last week.

That is used for people or things. *That* is usually informal when used to describe people.

Example: Is this the only book *that Louis L'Amour wrote?*

Example: Is Louis L'Amour the author *that wrote Western novels?*

Who is used for people or for animals that have an identity or personality.

Example: Mozart was the composer *who wrote those operas.*

Example: John's dog, *who is called Max,* is large and fierce.

Then and Than

Then is an adverb that indicates sequence or order:

Example: I'm going to run to the library and then come home.

Than is special-purpose word used only for comparisons:

Example: Susie likes chips more than candy.

Saw and Seen

Saw is the past-tense form of *see.*

Example: I saw a turtle on my walk this morning.

Seen is the past participle of *see.*

Example: I have seen this movie before.

Affect and Effect

There are two main reasons that *affect* and *effect* are so often confused: 1) both words can be used as either a noun or a verb, and 2) unlike most homophones, their usage and meanings are closely related to each other. Here is a quick rundown of the four usage options:

Affect (n): feeling, emotion, or mood that is displayed

Example: The patient had a flat *affect.* (i.e., his face showed little or no emotion)

Affect (v): to alter, to change, to influence

Example: The sunshine *affects* the plant's growth.

Effect (n): a result, a consequence

Example: What *effect* will this weather have on our schedule?

Effect (v): to bring about, to cause to be

Example: These new rules will *effect* order in the office.

The noun form of *affect* is rarely used outside of technical medical descriptions, so if a noun form is needed on the test, you can safely select *effect*. The verb form of *effect* is not as rare as the noun form of *affect*, but it's still not all that likely to show up on your test. If you need a verb and you can't decide which to use based on the definitions, choosing *affect* is your best bet.

Homophones

Homophones are words that sound alike (or similar) but have different **spellings** and **definitions**. A homophone is a type of **homonym**, which is a pair or group of words that are pronounced or spelled the same, but do not mean the same thing.

To, Too, and Two

To can be an adverb or a preposition for showing direction, purpose, and relationship. See your dictionary for the many other ways to use *to* in a sentence.

Examples: I went to the store. | I want to go with you.

Too is an adverb that means *also, as well, very,* or *in excess.*

Examples: I can walk a mile too. | You have eaten too much.

Two is a number.

Example: You have two minutes left.

There, Their, and They're

There can be an adjective, adverb, or pronoun. Often, *there* is used to show a place or to start a sentence.

Examples: I went there yesterday. | There is something in his pocket.

Their is a pronoun that is used to show ownership.

Examples: He is their father. | This is their fourth apology this week.

They're is a contraction of *they are.*

Example: Did you know that they're in town?

Knew and New

Knew is the past tense of *know.*

Example: I knew the answer.

New is an adjective that means something is current, has not been used, or is modern.

Example: This is my new phone.

Its and It's

Its is a pronoun that shows ownership.

Example: The guitar is in its case.

It's is a contraction of *it is.*

Example: It's an honor and a privilege to meet you.

Note: The *h* in honor is silent, so *honor* starts with the vowel sound *o*, which must have the article *an*.

Your and You're

Your is a pronoun that shows ownership.

Example: This is your moment to shine.

You're is a contraction of *you are.*

Example: Yes, you're correct.

Homographs

Homographs are words that share the same spelling, but have different meanings and sometimes different pronunciations. To figure out which meaning is being used, you should be looking for context clues. The context clues give hints to the meaning of the word. For example, the word *spot* has many meanings. It can mean "a place" or "a stain or blot." In the sentence "After my lunch, I saw a spot on my shirt," the word *spot* means "a stain or blot." The context clues of "After my lunch" and "on my shirt" guide you to this decision. A homograph is another type of homonym.

Bank

(noun): an establishment where money is held for savings or lending

(verb): to collect or pile up

Content

(noun): the topics that will be addressed within a book

(adjective): pleased or satisfied

(verb): to make someone pleased or satisfied

Fine

(noun): an amount of money that acts a penalty for an offense

(adjective): very small or thin

(adverb): in an acceptable way

(verb): to make someone pay money as a punishment

Incense

(noun): a material that is burned in religious settings and makes a pleasant aroma

(verb): to frustrate or anger

Lead

(noun): the first or highest position

(noun): a heavy metallic element

(verb): to direct a person or group of followers

(adjective): containing lead

Object

(noun): a lifeless item that can be held and observed

(verb): to disagree

Produce

(noun): fruits and vegetables

(verb): to make or create something

Refuse

(noun): garbage or debris that has been thrown away

(verb): to not allow

Subject

(noun): an area of study

(verb): to force or subdue

Tear

(noun): a fluid secreted by the eyes

(verb): to separate or pull apart

Commonly Misused Words and Phrases

A Lot

The phrase *a lot* should always be written as two words; never as *alot*.

Correct: That's a lot of chocolate!

Incorrect: He does that alot.

CAN

The word *can* is used to describe things that are possible occurrences; the word *may* is used to described things that are allowed to happen.

Correct: May I have another piece of pie?

Correct: I can lift three of these bags of mulch at a time.

Incorrect: Mom said we can stay up thirty minutes later tonight.

COULD HAVE

The phrase *could of* is often incorrectly substituted for the phrase *could have*. Similarly, *could of*, *may of*, and *might of* are sometimes used in place of the correct phrases *could have*, *may have*, and *might have*.

Correct: If I had known, I would have helped out.

Incorrect: Well, that could of gone much worse than it did.

MYSELF

The word *myself* is a reflexive pronoun, often incorrectly used in place of *I* or *me*.

Correct: He let me do it myself.

Incorrect: The job was given to Dave and myself.

OFF

The phrase *off of* is a redundant expression that should be avoided. In most cases, it can be corrected simply by removing *of*.

Correct: My dog chased the squirrel off its perch on the fence.

Incorrect: He finally moved his plate off of the table.

SUPPOSED TO

The phrase *suppose to* is sometimes used incorrectly in place of the phrase *supposed to*.

Correct: I was supposed to go to the store this afternoon.

Incorrect: When are we suppose to get our grades?

TRY TO

The phrase *try and* is often used in informal writing and conversation to replace the correct phrase *try to*.

Correct: It's a good policy to try to satisfy every customer who walks in the door.

Incorrect: Don't try and do too much.

Spelling Conventions

General Spelling Rules

Words Ending with a Consonant

Usually, the final consonant is **doubled** on a word before adding a suffix. This is the rule for single syllable words, words ending with one consonant, and multi-syllable words with the last syllable accented. The following are examples:

- *beg* becomes *begging* (single syllable)
- *shop* becomes *shopped* (single syllable)
- *add* becomes *adding* (already ends in double consonant, do not add another *d*)
- *deter* becomes *deterring* (multi-syllable, accent on last syllable)
- *regret* becomes *regrettable* (multi-syllable, accent on last syllable)
- *compost* becomes *composting* (do not add another *t* because the accent is on the first syllable)

Words Ending with Y or C

The general rule for words ending in *y* is to keep the *y* when adding a suffix if the **y is preceded by a vowel**. If the word **ends in a consonant and y** the *y* is changed to an *i* before the suffix is added (unless the suffix itself begins with *i*). The following are examples:

- *pay* becomes *paying* (keep the *y*)
- *bully* becomes *bullied* (change to *i*)
- *bully* becomes *bullying* (keep the *y* because the suffix is *–ing*)

If a word ends with *c* and the suffix begins with an *e, i,* or *y*, the letter *k* is usually added to the end of the word. The following are examples:

- panic becomes panicky
- mimic becomes mimicking

Words Containing IE or EI, and/or Ending with E

Most words are spelled with an *i* before *e*, except when they follow the letter *c,* **or** sound like *a*. For example, the following words are spelled correctly according to these rules:

- piece, friend, believe (*i* before *e*)
- receive, ceiling, conceited (except after *c*)
- weight, neighborhood, veil (sounds like *a*)

To add a suffix to words ending with the letter *e*, first determine if the *e* is silent. If it is, the *e* will be kept if the added suffix begins with a consonant. If the suffix begins with a vowel, the *e* is dropped. The following are examples:

- *age* becomes *ageless* (keep the *e*)
- *age* becomes *aging* (drop the *e*)

An exception to this rule occurs when the word ends in *ce* or *ge* and the suffix *able* or *ous* is added; these words will retain the letter *e*. The following are examples:

- courage becomes courageous
- notice becomes noticeable

Words Ending with ISE or IZE

A small number of words end with *ise*. Most of the words in the English language with the same sound end in *ize*. The following are examples:

- advertise, advise, arise, chastise, circumcise, and comprise
- compromise, demise, despise, devise, disguise, enterprise, excise, and exercise
- franchise, improvise, incise, merchandise, premise, reprise, and revise
- supervise, surmise, surprise, and televise

Words that end with *ize* include the following:

- accessorize, agonize, authorize, and brutalize
- capitalize, caramelize, categorize, civilize, and demonize
- downsize, empathize, euthanize, idolize, and immunize
- legalize, metabolize, mobilize, organize, and ostracize
- plagiarize, privatize, utilize, and visualize

(Note that some words may technically be spelled with *ise*, especially in British English, but it is more common to use *ize*. Examples include *symbolize/symbolise* and *baptize/baptise*.)

Words Ending with CEED, SEDE, or CEDE

There are only three words in the English language that end with *ceed*: *exceed, proceed,* and *succeed*. There is only one word in the English language that ends with *sede*: *supersede*. Most other words that sound like *sede* or *ceed* end with *cede*. The following are examples:

- concede, recede, and precede

Words Ending in ABLE or IBLE

For words ending in *able* or *ible*, there are no hard and fast rules. The following are examples:

- adjustable, unbeatable, collectable, deliverable, and likeable
- edible, compatible, feasible, sensible, and credible

There are more words ending in *able* than *ible*; this is useful to know if guessing is necessary.

Words Ending in ANCE or ENCE

The suffixes *ence, ency,* and *ent* are used in the following cases:

- the suffix is preceded by the letter *c* but sounds like *s* – *innocence*
- the suffix is preceded by the letter *g* but sounds like *j* – *intelligence, negligence*

The suffixes *ance, ancy,* and *ant* are used in the following cases:

- the suffix is preceded by the letter *c* but sounds like *k* – *significant, vacant*
- the suffix is preceded by the letter *g* with a hard sound – *elegant, extravagance*

If the suffix is preceded by other letters, there are no clear rules. For example: *finance, abundance,* and *assistance* use the letter *a,* while *decadence, competence,* and *excellence* use the letter *e*.

Words Ending in tion, sion, or cian

Words ending in *tion, sion,* or *cian* all sound like *shun* or *zhun*. There are no rules for which ending is used for words. The following are examples:

- action, agitation, caution, fiction, nation, and motion
- admission, expression, mansion, permission, and television
- electrician, magician, musician, optician, and physician (note that these words tend to describe occupations)

Words with the ai or ia Combination

When deciding if *ai* or *ia* is correct, the combination of *ai* usually sounds like one vowel sound, as in *Britain*, while the vowels in *ia* are pronounced separately, as in *guardian*. The following are examples:

- captain, certain, faint, hair, malaise, and praise (*ai* makes one sound)
- bacteria, beneficiary, diamond, humiliation, and nuptial (*ia* makes two sounds)

Rules for Plurals

Nouns Ending in ch, sh, s, x, or z

When a noun ends in the letters *ch, sh, s, x,* or *z*, an *es* instead of a singular *s* is added to the end of the word to make it plural. The following are examples:

- church becomes churches
- bush becomes bushes
- bass becomes basses
- mix becomes mixes
- buzz becomes buzzes

This is the rule with proper names as well; the Ross family would become the Rosses.

Nouns Ending in y or ay/ey/iy/oy/uy

If a noun ends with a **consonant and y**, the plural is formed by replacing the *y* with *ies*. For example, *fly* becomes *flies* and *puppy* becomes *puppies*. If a noun ends with a **vowel and *y***, the plural is formed by adding an *s*. For example, *alley* becomes *alleys* and *boy* becomes *boys*.

Nouns Ending in f or fe

Most nouns ending in *f* or *fe* are pluralized by replacing the *f* with *v* and adding *es*. The following are examples:

- knife becomes knives; self becomes selves; wolf becomes wolves.

An exception to this rule is the word *roof; roof* becomes *roofs*.

Nouns Ending in o

Most nouns ending with a **consonant and *o*** are pluralized by adding *es*. The following are examples:

- hero becomes heroes; tornado becomes tornadoes; potato becomes potatoes

Most nouns ending with a **vowel and *o*** are pluralized by adding *s*. The following are examples:

- portfolio becomes portfolios; radio becomes radios; cameo becomes cameos.

An exception to these rules is seen with musical terms ending in *o*. These words are pluralized by adding *s* even if they end in a consonant and *o*. The following are examples: *soprano* becomes *sopranos; banjo* becomes *banjos; piano* becomes *pianos.*

Letters, Numbers, and Symbols

Letters and numbers become plural by adding an apostrophe and *s*. The following are examples:

- The *L's* are the people whose names begin with the letter *L*.
- They broke the teams down into groups of *3's*.
- The sorority girls were all *KD's*.

Compound Nouns

A **compound noun** is a noun that is made up of two or more words; they can be written with hyphens. For example, *mother-in-law* or *court-martial* are compound nouns. To make them plural, an *s* or *es* is added to the noun portion of the word. The following are examples: *mother-in-law* becomes *mothers-in-law; court-martial* becomes *courts-martial.*

Exceptions

Some words do not fall into any specific category for making the singular form plural. They are **irregular**. Certain words become plural by changing the vowels within the word. The following are examples:

- woman becomes women; goose becomes geese; foot becomes feet

Some words change in unusual ways in the plural form. The following are examples:

- mouse becomes mice; ox becomes oxen; person becomes people

Some words are the same in both the singular and plural forms. The following are examples:

- *Salmon*, *deer*, and *moose* are the same whether singular or plural.

Commonly Misspelled Words

accidentally	accommodate	accompanied	accompany
achieved	acknowledgment	across	address
aggravate	aisle	ancient	anxiety
apparently	appearance	arctic	argument
arrangement	attendance	auxiliary	awkward
bachelor	barbarian	beggar	beneficiary
biscuit	brilliant	business	cafeteria
calendar	campaign	candidate	ceiling
cemetery	changeable	changing	characteristic
chauffeur	colonel	column	commit
committee	comparative	compel	competent
competition	conceive	congratulations	conqueror
conscious	coolly	correspondent	courtesy
curiosity	cylinder	deceive	deference

deferred	definite	describe	desirable
desperate	develop	diphtheria	disappear
disappoint	disastrous	discipline	discussion
disease	dissatisfied	dissipate	drudgery
ecstasy	efficient	eighth	eligible
embarrass	emphasize	especially	exaggerate
exceed	exhaust	exhilaration	existence
explanation	extraordinary	familiar	fascinate
February	fiery	finally	forehead
foreign	foreigner	foremost	forfeit
ghost	glamorous	government	grammar
grateful	grief	grievous	handkerchief
harass	height	hoping	hurriedly
hygiene	hypocrisy	imminent	incidentally
incredible	independent	indigestible	inevitable
innocence	intelligible	intentionally	intercede
interest	irresistible	judgment	legitimate
liable	library	likelihood	literature
maintenance	maneuver	manual	mathematics
mattress	miniature	mischievous	misspell
momentous	mortgage	neither	nickel
niece	ninety	noticeable	notoriety
obedience	obstacle	occasion	occurrence
omitted	operate	optimistic	organization
outrageous	pageant	pamphlet	parallel
parliament	permissible	perseverance	persuade
physically	physician	possess	possibly
practically	prairie	preceding	prejudice
prevalent	professor	pronunciation	pronouncement
propeller	protein	psychiatrist	psychology
quantity	questionnaire	rally	recede
receive	recognize	recommend	referral
referred	relieve	religious	resistance
restaurant	rhetoric	rhythm	ridiculous
sacrilegious	salary	scarcely	schedule
secretary	sentinel	separate	severely
sheriff	shriek	similar	soliloquy
sophomore	species	strenuous	studying
suffrage	supersede	suppress	surprise
symmetry	temperament	temperature	tendency
tournament	tragedy	transferred	truly
twelfth	tyranny	unanimous	unpleasant
usage	vacuum	valuable	vein
vengeance	vigilance	villain	Wednesday
weird	wholly		

Chapter Quiz

Ready to see how well you retained what you just read? Scan the QR code to go directly to the chapter quiz interface for this study guide. If you're using a computer, simply visit the online resources page at **mometrix.com/resources719/pnat** and click the Chapter Quizzes link.

P-NAT Practice Test

Want to take this practice test in an online interactive format?
Check out the online resources page, which includes interactive practice questions and much more: **mometrix.com/resources719/pnat**

Reading Comprehension/Reasoning Ability

Read the following passage carefully. Answer questions 1–10 following the passage based on the information in the passage by choosing the correct answer from the four choices given. Work quickly but carefully.

It was moving day for the Robertson family. Bernard and Marian had married before World War II. Bernard was in the Army. When he returned from his tour of duty, the couple lived with Marian's widowed mother in the house her late husband had left to her. After several years they had a son, Lewis. Two years later they had a daughter, Hannah. When the children were seven and five years old respectively, their parents had both worked and saved up enough money to have a new house built. Now they were finally moving in, bringing along Marian's mother, whom the children called Nana, and their pet cat, whom they had named Fluffy.

The house was not completely finished, but it was livable. It was a hot summer day. After hours of setting up their furniture brought by the movers, and bringing in and unpacking many belongings, the family sat down to take a breather. Suddenly they noticed that Fluffy was missing. Fearing he had run outside during all the moving commotion and become lost in a new neighborhood, Marian and Hannah went walking around the block, calling their pet's name. Marian had contracted a terrible case of poison oak on her legs from petting Katie, a neighbor's beautiful Irish setter who had picked up the poison oak oils on her coat from running through the woods and then rubbed against Marian's bare legs. This made it painful for her to walk in the summer heat, but she was so worried about Fluffy. Hannah was equally distressed about her beloved pet.

After searching to no avail, the family decided to sit down to eat dinner and hope that Fluffy would show up at some point. Right in the middle of the meal, they heard a "Meow!" coming from the adjacent living room. Turning to look in the direction of the sound, they spotted Fluffy sitting on the hearth of their new fireplace! Excited, they all jumped up, shouting, "Fluffy!" Upon hearing the clamor, the little tabby immediately turned and jumped up into the chimney to escape. Now they realized that he had not been lost or outdoors at all, but had simply found a dark, quiet, cool place to hide from the commotion. Reaching up into the chimney, Bernard and Lewis discovered a ledge where Fluffy was comfortably perched. Marian offered up a little dish of hamburger, a favorite treat; but Fluffy just ate the meat without emerging from his hiding place. The family all laughed together at the kitty's cleverness and Mom's foolishness in not placing the meat farther away to lure him out of hiding.

The family agreed that it would be best to give their pet the safety and seclusion he needed after all the trauma of moving (cats generally hate any changes in their environment), and the noise and confusion of things being brought in and moved about, people coming in and going out, and so forth. They let him stay in the chimney. Once things had settled down and it was quiet in the house, Fluffy eventually came out of his safe refuge and began to explore his new surroundings. Soon he had adjusted to the new home. He slept on Hannah's bed, lounged on the living room chairs, kept Nana company while she sewed when the parents were at work and the children were at school, and scampered around the house playing. He had completely gotten over his initial fear and made himself at home with his family.

1. This story takes place:

a. Several years after World War I.
b. Several years after World War II.
c. Several years after the Korean War.
d. This information is not given in the story.

2. Nana was:

a. What the children called their mother.
b. The name the family gave to their cat.
c. What the kids called their grandmother.
d. The nickname the family called Hannah.

3. Marian contracted poison oak from:

a. Running through the neighborhood woods.
b. Petting their cat Fluffy who had it on his coat.
c. Walking around the block in the summer heat.
d. Having the dog Katie rub against her bare legs.

4. Before building their first new home, the Robertson family lived:

a. In Nana's house.
b. In an apartment.
c. In another town.
d. This is not given.

5. The "tour of duty" referred to in the passage means:

a. The term that a soldier serves in the armed forces.
b. A program of visiting various countries in the world.
c. Fulfilling all the duties of moving into a new house.
d. There is no such reference existing in this passage.

6. How did the family discover where Fluffy had been?

a. He came to the dinner table, lured by the smell of meat.
b. During dinner, they heard him meow from the living room.
c. After hearing him, they saw him go back up the chimney.
d. They walked around the block calling until they found him.

7. Why was Fluffy sitting on a ledge inside the chimney?

a. Cats just naturally always hide.
b. It was cooler on a summer day.
c. To escape all the commotion.
d. Both (B) and (C) are correct.

8. Which is the *least likely* reason Fluffy found moving day traumatic?

a. Cats hate any changes in their environment.
b. The moving process is noisy and confusing.
c. There was a dog in the new neighborhood.
d. It kept him from feeling privacy and safety.

9. Which of the following is NOT included among Fluffy's activities once he adjusted?

a. Lounging on living room chairs
b. Keeping Nana company sewing
c. Climbing drapes in Lewis's room
d. Sleeping in Hannah's bedroom

10. The main focus of this passage is:

a. How the family lived with the grandmother in both homes.
b. How hard two parents worked and saved to build a house.
c. How difficult it was to move the family into the new home.
d. How a family "lost" and then found their cat when moving.

Read the following passage carefully. Answer questions 11–20 following the passage based on the information in the passage by choosing the correct answer from the four choices given. Work quickly but carefully.

The phrase "boulevard of broken dreams" may be familiar to many people, because it has been used so often. In 1933, the songwriting team of lyricist Al Dubin and composer Harry Warren wrote a song entitled "Boulevard of Broken Dreams," which was a big hit in its day and, a version sung by Constance Bennett was included in the 1934 movie *Moulin Rouge.* The lyrics include the verses, "I walk along the street of sorrow/The Boulevard of Broken Dreams/Where gigolo and gigolette/Can take a kiss without regret/So they forget their broken dreams....Here is where you'll always find me/Always walking up and down...." Many other singers have covered this song over the years, including a 2006 duet by Tony Bennett and Sting, and some as recently as 2010 and 2012. The phrase "boulevard of broken dreams" was a reference to Sunset Boulevard in Los Angeles.

In 1942, the modern American artist Edward Hopper created an oil painting he called *Nighthawks.* It depicts a late-night scene of a diner in a downtown area. The street outside is deserted, and inside the lighted diner are three customers sitting at the counter and a man with a white hat and shirt behind the counter. This painting became very famous. What does this painting have to do with the phrase "boulevard of broken dreams"? Well, contemporary Viennese artist Gottfried Helnwein (born in 1948) created a parody of Hopper's painting in 1984. Helnwein's watercolor appears quite similar to Hopper's work—until you look more closely. Then you see that the anonymous people sitting in the diner in Hopper's original have been replaced in Helnwein's version with the iconic late celebrity actors Humphrey

Bogart, Marilyn Monroe, and James Dean; and the attendant behind the counter has been replaced with the late Elvis Presley. These famous figures had all died young between 1955 and 1977.

Helnwein's was one of a number of parodies based on Hopper's painting. It inspired Billie Joe Armstrong, the lyricist and lead singer of the contemporary rock band Green Day, to write a song entitled "Boulevard of Broken Dreams." Its music and lyrics are different from the 1933 song: "I walk a lonely road/The only one that I have ever known/Don't know where it goes/But it's home to me and I walk alone/I walk alone, I walk alone…I walk this empty street/On the Boulevard of Broken Dreams/When the city sleeps/And I'm the only one and I walk alone/My shadow's the only one that walks beside me/My shallow heart's the only thing that's beating/Sometimes I wish someone up there will find me/'til then I walk alone." Released in 2004 on their album *American Idiot,* the song became one of Green Day's biggest and most recognized hits.

Green Day was not the only example of works using the title "Boulevard of Broken Dreams." Country singer Ferlin Husky released an album with that title in 1957. The band Smokie released both an album and its title song with the same name in 1989. Songs with this title were also recorded by Juan García Esquivel (1958), Hanoi Rocks (1984), Brian Setzer (1986), David Cassidy (1990), Beatmasters (1991), and with the same title in Spanish by Joaquín Sabina (1994). In addition to painters and musicians, other artists have used the familiar phrase. Science fiction author Harlan Ellison entitled a 1978 short story "Boulevard of Broken Dreams," which he published in *Strange Wine,* a collection of his stories. An Australian movie with this title was released in 1988. Paul Alexander published a biography of James Dean entitled *Boulevard of Broken Dreams* (1994)—perhaps inspired by Dean's likeness in Helnwein's painting. Kim Deitch published an acclaimed graphic novel (2002) with the same title. In 2007, the E! television network aired a documentary series about celebrities, also using this title.

11. The earliest use of the title and lyric "Boulevard of Broken Dreams" identified in the passage was by:

a. Billie Joe Armstrong
b. Tony Bennett and Sting
c. Al Dubin and Harry Warren
d. Gottfried Helnwein

12. The famous painting by Edward Hopper described in the passage is entitled:

a. Boulevard of Broken Dreams
b. American Idiot
c. Strange Wine
d. Nighthawks

13. In the movie *Moulin Rouge,* a song entitled "Boulevard of Broken Dreams" is sung by:

a. Constance Bennett
b. Tony Bennett and Sting
c. Billie Joe and Green Day
d. Juan García Esquivel

14. Which is correct about the media used by two painters described in the passage?

a. Hopper used watercolors, and Helnwein used oils.
b. Hopper used oils, and Helnwein used watercolors.
c. Both Hopper and Helnwein used oils in their work.
d. Both Hopper and Helnwein used watercolor paint.

15. According to the passage, who wrote the lyrics "I walk alone, I walk alone"?

a. Al Dubin
b. Harry Warren
c. Constance Bennett
d. Billie Joe Armstrong

16. Which celebrities are portrayed in Edward Hopper's famous painting?

a. James Dean
b. Elvis Presley
c. Marilyn Monroe
d. None of these.

17. Related to "Boulevard of Broken Dreams," which of the following occurred earliest in time?

a. Paul Alexander wrote a biography of James Dean with this title.
b. Kim Deitch published an acclaimed graphic novel using this title.
c. Harlan Ellison published a science fiction story that had the title.
d. E! television network aired a documentary series with this title.

18. Green Day's hit song was inspired by:

a. The famous painting by Edward Hopper.
b. The Hopper parody by Gottfried Helnwein.
c. The 1933 song by Al Dubin and Harry Warren.
d. The movie *Moulin Rouge*, first released in 1934.

19. The title "Boulevard of Broken Dreams" has been used in:

a. Paintings, songs, albums, movies, books, and TV.
b. Many individual songs, but never in any albums.
c. Movies and a TV series, but never in any books.
d. Paintings and songs, but never in books or TV.

20. The celebrities depicted in the painting described:

a. Had all been dead for years when the painting was made.
b. Had all just recently died when the painting was created.
c. Were all still alive at the time the artist made the painting.
d. Cannot be determined as dead or alive from this passage.

Directions for questions 21–30

Read the statement or passage and then choose the best answer to the question. Answer the question based on what is stated or implied in the statement or passage.

21. During the 1970s, a new type of pet became popular in North America. Although they were actually just brine shrimp, they were marketed as "Sea Monkeys." They don't actually look like monkeys at all, but were branded as such due to their long tails. When sea monkeys first began to be sold in the United States, they were sold under the brand name "Instant Life." Later, when they became known as sea monkeys, the cartoon drawings that were featured in comic books showed creatures that resembled humans more than shrimp. The creative marketing of these creatures can only be described as genius, and at the height of their popularity in the 1970s, they could be found in as many as one in five homes.

Based on the information in the passage, it can be inferred that

a. Sea monkeys were more popular when they were marketed as "instant life."
b. Sea monkeys wouldn't have been as popular if they had been marketed as "brine shrimp."
c. Most people thought they were actually purchasing monkeys that lived in the sea.
d. There are more homes today that have sea monkeys than there were in the 1970s.

22. Before the battle between CDs and MP3s, there was a rivalry during the 1960s between the four-track and the eight-track tape. Four-track tapes were invented in the early 1960s by Earl Muntz, an entrepreneur from California. Later, Bill Lear designed the eight-track tape. This latter invention was similar in size to the four-track tape, but it could store and play twice as many songs. Lear had close ties with the motor company Ford, and he convinced them to include eight-track players in their vehicles, which definitely helped the eight-track tape to achieve a high level of popularity. Soon after, they began being used in homes, and the four-track tape all but disappeared.

The main difference between the four-track and eight-track tape was

a. The four-track tape was much larger than the eight-track tape.
b. The eight-track tape cost a lot more to produce than the four-track tape.
c. The eight-track tape could hold more songs than the four-track tape.
d. The four-track tape was usually included in Ford vehicles.

23. It is natural for humans to have fears, but when those fears are completely irrational and begin to interfere with everyday activities they are known as phobias. Agoraphobia is a serious phobia, and it can be devastating for those who suffer from it. Contrary to popular belief, agoraphobia is not simply a fear of open spaces. Rather, the agoraphobic fears being in a place that he feels is unsafe. Depending on the severity of the problem, the agoraphobic might fear going to the mall, walking down the street, or even walking to the mailbox. Often, the agoraphobic will view his home as the safest possible place to be, and he may even be reluctant to leave his house. Treatments for this condition include medication and behavioral therapy.

An agoraphobic would feel safest

a. In their yard.
b. In their house.
c. In a mall.
d. On the sidewalk.

24. The butterfly effect is a somewhat poorly understood mathematical concept, primarily because it is interpreted and presented incorrectly by the popular media. It refers to systems and how initial conditions can influence the ultimate outcome of an event. The best way to understand the concept is through an example. You have two rubber balls. There are two inches between them, and you release them. Where will they end up? Well, that depends. If they're in a sloped, sealed container, they will end up two inches away from each other at the end of the slope. If it's the top of a mountain, however, they may end up miles away from each other. They could bounce off rocks; one could get stuck in a snow bank while the other continues down the slope; one could enter a river and get swept away. The fact that even a tiny initial difference can have a significant overall impact is known as the butterfly effect.

The purpose of this passage is

a. To discuss what could happen to two rubber balls released on top of a mountain.
b. To show why you can predict what will happen to two objects in a sloped, sealed container.
c. To discuss the primary reason why the butterfly effect is a poorly understood concept.
d. To give an example of how small changes at the beginning of an event can have large effects.

25. Wells provide water for drinking, bathing, and cleaning to many people across the world. When wells are being dug, there are several issues that must be taken into account to minimize the chance of potential problems down the road. First, it's important to be aware that groundwater levels differ, depending on the season. In general, groundwater levels will be higher during the winter. So if a well is being dug during the winter, it should be deep enough to remain functional during the summer when water levels are lower. Well water that is used is replaced by melting snow and rain. If the well owners are using the water faster than it can be replaced, however, the water levels will be lowered. The only way to remedy this, aside from waiting for the groundwater to be replenished naturally, is to deepen the well.

From this passage, it can be concluded that

a. It is better to have a well that is too deep than one that is too shallow.
b. Most well owners will face significant water shortages every year.
c. Most people who dig wells during the winter do not make them deep enough.
d. Well water is safe to use for bathing and cleaning, but it is not suitable for drinking.

26. Today's low-fat craze has led many people to assume that all fats are unhealthy, but this is simply not the case. Fat is an essential component of any healthy diet because it provides energy and helps the body process nutrients. While all fats should be consumed in moderation, there are good and bad fats. Good fats are what are known as unsaturated fats. They are found in olive oil, fatty fish like salmon, and nuts. Bad fats are saturated and trans fats. They are found in foods like butter, bacon, and ice cream. Consumption of foods that contain trans or saturated fats should be restricted or avoided altogether.

The main purpose of this passage is to

a. Explain why fat is important for the body.
b. Discuss some of the main sources of good fats.
c. Talk about the different types of fats.
d. Discuss examples of foods that should be avoided.

27. Satire is a genre that originated in the ancient world and is still popular today. Although satire is often humorous, its purposes and intentions go well beyond simply making people laugh. Satire is a way for the playwright, author, or television producer to criticize society, human nature, and individuals that he holds in contempt. Satire as we know it today developed in Ancient Greece and Rome. There were three main types. The first, Menippean satire, focused on criticizing aspects of human nature. This was done by introducing stereotypical, one-dimensional characters. Horatian satire can be viewed as gentle satire. It made fun of people and their habits, but in a way that was not offensive. Juvenalian satire was written is such a way that the audience would experience feelings of disgust and aversion when they saw the characters and their actions. Some of the most popular satires today are fake news shows, like the *Daily Show* and the *Colbert Report*, and satirical comic strips like *Doonesbury*.

The main purpose of the passage is

a. To discuss the history of satire.
b. To present the major types of satire.
c. To discuss modern examples of satire.
d. To present the purposes of satire.

28. Many people believe that how we express our feelings is mainly determined by our upbringing and culture. Undoubtedly, this is true in some cases. In North America, for example, it is customary to shake hands when we meet somebody to express acceptance, whereas in other countries they may simply bow slightly to indicate this. Many feelings, however, are expressed in similar ways by people all over the world. These emotions include, fear, anger, happiness, disgust, and sorrow. For example, if a person is experiencing fear, their eyes will widen and their pupils will dilate. This reaction is largely involuntary. The finding that people express many feelings in a similar manner, regardless of where they are from, indicates that facial expressions are influenced more by evolution than culture.

Based on the passage, it can be concluded that

a. People often can't hide what they are feeling.
b. People from other parts of the world express happiness differently.
c. Fear is the only emotion that is felt by everybody in the world.
d. Acceptance is a feeling invented by man.

29. Cities are typically warmer than the surrounding countryside, a phenomenon known as the heat island effect. There are numerous causes of this phenomenon, including emissions from cars and buildings. This creates a mini greenhouse effect. In rural areas, the standing water in marshes and ponds evaporates, which cools the air slightly. This does not occur to the same extent in the city. The tall buildings in the center of most cities block winds that would provide some relief from the excessive heat. Finally, the color and material of most roads and buildings absorbs rather than reflects heat. Although planting trees and using building materials that reflect heat may alleviate the problem somewhat, it will by no means eliminate it.

The main purpose of the passage is to

a. Talk about how the problem of heat island can be solved.
b. Argue that cities should make an effort to plant more trees.
c. Present the major causes of the problem of heat island.
d. Contrast the city environment to that of the countryside.

30. Marsupials resemble mammals in a number of ways. For one thing, they are warm-blooded creatures. They have hair, and the mothers feed their young by producing milk. However, one thing that separates marsupials from mammals is that their young are born when they are not yet fully-developed. Most are born after only about four or five weeks. They finish their development in the pouch of their mother. Some of the more commonly known marsupials are koalas, kangaroos, and opossums. They are a diverse group, with many members having little in common besides their reproductive traits.

A major difference between marsupials and mammals is

a. Marsupials have hair, while mammals do not.
b. Mammals are a much more diverse group than marsupials.
c. Marsupials are born at an earlier stage of development.
d. Mammals feed their young by producing milk.

Directions for questions 31–40

For the questions that follow, two underlined sentences are followed by a question or statement. Read the sentences, then choose the best answer to the question or the best completion of the statement.

31. Atheists are individuals who do not believe in any type of higher power.

Theists usually possess religious and spiritual beliefs and have faith in one or more gods.

What does the second sentence do?

a. It states an example.
b. It makes a contrast.
c. It disputes the first sentence.
d. It offers a solution.

32. Home schooling refers to the practice of educating children at home rather than sending them to school.

Home schooling usually involves one parent giving up their career in order to stay home.

What does the second sentence do?

a. It restates the information from the first.
b. It provides an example.
c. It states an effect.
d. It contradicts the first.

33. Coffee is the most popular beverage in the entire world, and it is estimated that about 80% of Americans drink coffee.

According to a recent study, about 85% of North Americans drink soda, making it the most popular drink worldwide.

What does the second sentence do?

a. It makes a contrast.
b. It gives an example.
c. It supports the first.
d. It contradicts the first.

34. Regeneration refers to the ability that some animals have to replace severed body parts.

A salamander that has had its tail chopped off can grow a new one that is practically identical to the original.

What does the second sentence do?

a. It restates the information from the first.
b. It provides an example.
c. It supports the first.
d. It presents a solution.

35. Even though monthly rent on an apartment is usually less than a mortgage payment, most people would still rather own their own home.

Home ownership is a dream for most North Americans, even though monthly costs for houses are higher than those for apartments.

What does the second sentence do?

a. It contradicts the first.
b. It supports the first.
c. It restates the information in the first.
d. It explains the information in the first.

36. Soil contamination can be caused by a wide variety of factors, including leakage from underground septic tanks.

Septic tanks will corrode over time, and when they leak or rupture, the contents contaminate the surrounding soil.

What does the second sentence do?

a. It expands on the first.
b. It restates the information in the first.
c. It states an effect.
d. It proposes a solution.

37. The Richter Scale is the most commonly-used method to measure the strength of earthquakes.

Even though other methods are used more frequently to measure earthquakes, the Richter Scale is the most trusted.

What does the second sentence do?

a. It provides an example.
b. It reinforces the information in the first.
c. It contradicts the information in the first.
d. It presents a conclusion.

38. Adaptation refers to the ability of an animal to change in order to be better suited for its environment and to increase its chances of survival.

Porcupines have sharp quills that can be used to ward off animals that might otherwise try to hunt them.

What does the second sentence do?

a. It expands on the information in the first.
b. It presents an example.
c. It states an effect.
d. It makes an inference.

39. Congestion due to excessive traffic means that many people are forced to sit in traffic on their way to work.

Carpooling and public transportation can effectively reduce the number of cars on the road.

How are the two sentences related?

a. They explain several concepts.
b. They provide a concept and an example.
c. They support one another.
d. They state a problem and a solution.

40. Men are known for being analytical when they make decisions.

Women often make decisions based on intuition and gut feelings.

What does the second sentence do?

a. It gives an example.
b. It expands on the first.
c. It provides a contrast.
d. It contradicts the first.

NUMERICAL ABILITY

1.

236
+301

a. 505
b. 507
c. 535
d. 537

2.

4,307
+1,864

a. 5,161
b. 5,271
c. 6,171
d. 6,271

3. If a=3 and b=-2, what is the value of $a^2+3ab-b^2$?

a. 5
b. -13
c. -4
d. -20

4.

356
-167

a. 189
b. 198
c. 211
d. 298

5.

5,306
-3,487

a. 1,181
b. 1,819
c. 2,119
d. 2,189

6. 324 is what percent of 80?

a. 25%
b. 32%
c. 40%
d. 44%

7.

$$\begin{array}{r} 707 \\ \times \underline{\ 17} \end{array}$$

a. 12,019
b. 12,049
c. 17,019
d. 17,049

8. $7\overline{)917}$

a. 131
b. 131 R4
c. 145
d. 145 R4

9. Factor the following expression: $x^2 + x - 12$

a. $(x - 4)\ (x + 4)$
b. $(x - 2)\ (x + 6)$
c. $(x + 6)\ (x - 2)$
d. $(x + 4)\ (x - 3)$

10. $\frac{38}{100}$ as a decimal

a. 0.38
b. 0.038
c. 3.8
d. 0.0038

11.

$$\begin{array}{r} 6.8 \\ 11.3 \\ + \underline{0.06} \end{array}$$

a. 17.16
b. 17.70
c. 18.16
d. 18.70

12. The average of six numbers is 4. If the average of two of those numbers is 2, what is the average of the other four numbers?

a. 5
b. 6
c. 7
d. 8

13. Which numeral is in the thousandths place in 0.3874?

a. 3
b. 8
c. 7
d. 4

14. 0.58 - 0.39=

a. 0.19
b. 1.9
c. 0.29
d. 2.9

15. Solve: 0.25 × 0.03 =

a. 75
b. 0.075
c. 0.75
d. 0.0075

16. $3\frac{1}{8} + 6 + \frac{3}{7} =$

a. 9 31/56
b. 9 1/2
c. 9 21/56
d. 9 7/8

17. $4\frac{1}{7} - 2\frac{1}{2} =$

a. 2 5/14
b. 1 5/14
c. 1 9/14
d. 2 9/14

18. $1\frac{1}{4} \times 3\frac{2}{5} \times 1\frac{2}{3} =$

a. 7 1/12
b. 5 5/6
c. 6 7/12
d. 8 11/15

19. How many 3-inch segments can a 4.5-yard line be divided into?

a. 15
b. 45
c. 54
d. 64

20. Reduce $\frac{14}{98}$ **to lowest terms.**

a. $\frac{7}{49}$
b. $\frac{2}{14}$
c. $\frac{1}{7}$
d. $\frac{3}{8}$

21. Thirty six hundredths as a percent.

a. 36%
b. 3.6%
c. 0.36%
d. 0.036%

22. 40% of 900

a. 280
b. 340
c. 360
d. 420

23. Sheila, Janice, and Karen, working together at the same rate, can complete a job in 3 1/3 days. Working at the same rate, how much of the job could Janice and Karen do in one day?

a. 1/5
b. 1/4
c. 1/3
d. 1/9

24. Three eighths of forty equals:

a. 15
b. 20
c. 22
d. 24

25. 6% of 25

a. .3
b. 1.5
c. 3.0
d. 15

26. Ratio of 4 to 16 = (?)%

a. 2
b. 4
c. 12
d. 25

27. $4^6 \div 2^8 =$

a. 2
b. 8
c. 16
d. 32

28. 30% as a reduced common fraction

a. 30/100
b. 1/30
c. 23/10
d. 3/10

29. 37% as a decimal

a. .0037
b. .037
c. .37
d. 3.7

30. $-4a + 6a + 2a$

a. $4a$
b. $-4a$
c. $8a$
d. $12a$

31. $18 + 7 - (-5) + 11 = ?$

a. 31
b. 41
c. 51
d. 21
e. 11

32. Luis left home with $5.50 in his wallet. He spent $3.25 on drinks and $2.00 on a magazine. Later, his friend repaid him $3.50 that he had borrowed the previous day. How much did Luis have in his wallet then?

a. $12.25
b. $14.25
c. $3.25
d. $3.75
e. $1.75

33. $\frac{1}{3} + \left(\frac{1}{5} \times \frac{2}{3}\right) - \left(\frac{2}{5} \times \frac{1}{3}\right) = ?$

a. $\frac{1}{3}$
b. $-\frac{1}{3}$
c. $\frac{2}{15}$
d. $-\frac{2}{15}$
e. $\frac{3}{15}$

34. John needed 13.71 feet of wire to fix a lamp. He bought $14\frac{1}{2}$ feet of wire at the hardware store. How much wire did he have left over after fixing the lamp?

a. $\frac{3}{4}$ ft
b. 0.29 ft
c. 0.81 ft
d. 1.29 ft
e. 0.79 ft

35. A music club offers 7 CDs for $24 to new members. The usual price of CDs is $12 each. If Maria joins the club and gets her 7 CDs at the discounted price instead of buying them individually, how much is her total savings?

a. $53
b. $24
c. $84
d. $60
e. $79

36. $\mathbf{7,600,000 - 24,000 = ?}$

a. 7.576×10^6
b. 7.36×10^6
c. 7.84×10^6
d. 7.576×10^5
e. 7.84×10^5

37. Which of the following expressions is equivalent to $3 < x^{\frac{1}{2}} < 5$ **?**

a. $3 < x < 5$
b. $3 < x < 15$
c. $9 < x < 15$
d. $9 < x < 25$
e. $3 < x < 25$

38. $\mathbf{3 \times \sqrt[3]{27} = ?}$

a. 3
b. 81
c. 27
d. 9
e. 8

39. What is the value of x if $\frac{7}{11} = \frac{x}{7}$**?**

a. 7
b. $\frac{49}{11}$
c. 77
d. 121
e. $\frac{11}{7}$

40. If 12 gallons of gasoline costs $48.75, what is the cost of 13 gallons of gasoline?

a. $50.25
b. $\frac{12}{13} \times \$48.75$
c. $\frac{13}{12} \times \$48.75$
d. $\frac{\$48.75}{12 \times 13}$
e. $\frac{12 \times 13}{\$48.75}$

41. Fifty-five people take a math exam. Eighty percent of them pass. How many people failed the exam?

a. 5.5
b. 10
c. 16
d. 44
e. 11

42. Three quarters of the participants in a bicycle race crossed the finish line in less than 3 hours. How many finished in less than 3 hours?

a. 25%
b. $\frac{3}{4}$%
c. 75%
d. 67%
e. 50%

43. Ricky took the SAT math test four times. The first three scores totaled 1,900. After fourth time, his average score was 650. What score did he get the fourth time?

a. 600
b. 650
c. 700
d. 750
e. 800

44. Three quarters of the students running a 100-yard race finished with an average time of 16 seconds. The remaining 25% of students finished with an average time of 12 seconds. What was the average time overall?

a. 13 seconds
b. 14 seconds
c. 15 seconds
d. 16 seconds
e. 17 seconds

45. Manuella makes $21 in commissions over the first three hours that she worked selling magazines. How many dollars must she make during the fourth hour to average $8 an hour for the full four hours?

a. $8
b. $11
c. $12
d. $15
e. $10

46. 6/12 is equivalent to which fraction?

a. 10/24
b. 3/4
c. 3/6
d. 1/6

47. 675 × 7 =

a. 4,535
b. 4,675
c. 4,865
d. 4,725

48. Which of the following is closest to 5,465 + 394?

a. 5,000
b. 5,500
c. 6,000
d. 6,500

49. 11/12 - 1/6 =

a. 1/4
b. 1/2
c. 3/4
d. 5/6

50. 743 – 87 =

a. 626
b. 656
c. 674
d. 694

Language Ability

1. <u>Generous</u> most nearly means

a. giving
b. truthful
c. selfish
d. harsh

2. The math test was quite <u>challenging.</u>

a. reasonable
b. lengthy
c. difficult
d. simple

3. <u>Instructor</u> most nearly means

a. pupil
b. teacher
c. survivor
d. dictator

4. The audience applauded after the woman <u>concluded</u> her presentation.

a. delivered
b. prepared
c. attended
d. finished

5. <u>Residence</u> most nearly means

a. home
b. area
c. plan
d. resist

6. The company <u>instantly</u> agreed to the terms of the contract.

a. reluctantly
b. eventually
c. immediately
d. definitely

7. <u>Gigantic</u> most nearly means

a. small
b. great
c. huge
d. scary

8. The new car was very <u>costly</u>.

a. expensive
c. cheap
c. attractive
d. rare

9. <u>Opportunity</u> most nearly means

a. event
b. plan
c. direction
d. chance

10. The woman's <u>response</u> to the question was correct.

a. hesitation
b. answer
c. decision
d. concern

11. <u>Frequently</u> most nearly means

a. difficulty
b. freely
c. often
d. easy

12. He <u>observed</u> the eagles with binoculars.

a. watched
b. hunted
c. scared
d. sold

13. <u>Purchased</u> most nearly means

a. sold
b. bargained
c. complained
d. bought

14. She is having <u>difficulties</u> with her new computer.

a. experiences
b. solutions
c. pleasures
d. problems

15. <u>Entire</u> most nearly means

a. whole
b. divide
c. tired
d. basic

16. The woman's performance was <u>superior</u> to the man's.

a. short
b. similar
c. better
d. weak

17. <u>Remark</u> most nearly means

a. rebuke
b. comment
c. lecture
d. replace

18. <u>Selecting</u> the best person for the job was difficult.

a. locating
b. contacting
c. choosing
d. informing

19. <u>Commence</u> most nearly means

a. begin
b. progress
c. finish
d. comment

20. The fox ran <u>swiftly</u> after its prey.

a. surely
b. quickly
c. slowly
d. lightly

Directions for questions 21–40

Each question gives three different spellings of a word. Two are incorrect and one is correct. Select the choice from each set of three that is spelled correctly.

21. A. separate	B. seperate	C. sepparate
22. A. nucular	B. nuclear	C. nuculear
23. A. fermiliar	B. farmiliar	C. familiar
24. A. sacrilegious	B. sacreligious	C. sacraligious
25. A. aggitated	B. agittated	C. agitated
26. A. orientated	B. oriented	C. oriented
27. A. indispensible	B. indespensible	C. indispensable
28. A. similar	B. simular	C. similar
29. A. atitude	B. attitude	C. attitude
30. A. abreviate	B. abbreviate	C. abreeviate
31. A. absorb	B. apsorb	C. absorb
32. A. acumulate	B. acummulate	C. accumulate
33. A. airial	B. aireal	C. aerial

34. A. comedian B. commedian C. comedien

35. A. ashphalt B. asphalt C. aspalt

36. A. forseable B. forcible C. forcible

37. A. anicdote B. antecdote C. anecdote

38. A. flexible B. flexable C. flexiable

39. A. defendant B. defendent C. difendent

40. A. plainteff B. plaintif C. plaintiff

Directions for questions 41–60

Select the best version of the underlined part of the sentence. The first choice is the same as the original sentence. If you think the original sentence is best, choose the first answer.

41. Several theories <u>about what caused dinosaurs to have extinction exist</u>, but scientists are still unable to reach a concrete conclusion.

a. about what caused dinosaurs to have extinction exist
b. about what caused dinosaurs to become extinct exist
c. about the causes of the dinosaur extinction exists
d. regarding the cause of extinction of dinosaurs exist

42. <u>Although most persons</u> prefer traditional pets like cats and dogs, others gravitate towards exotic animals like snakes and lizards.

a. Although most persons
b. Because most people
c. While most people
d. Maybe some persons

43. It is important that software companies offer tech support <u>to customers who are encountering problems</u>.

a. to customers who are encountering problems
b. because not all customers encounter problems
c. with customers who encounter problems
d. to customer who is encountering difficulties

44. The fact that children eat high fat diets and watch excessive amount of television are a cause of concern for many parents.

a. that children eat high fat diets and watch excessive amount of television are a cause of concern
b. the children eat high fat diets and watches excessive amount of television are a cause of concern
c. is children eat high fat diets and watch excessive amount of television is a cause for concern
d. that children eat high fat diets and watch excessive amounts of television is a cause for concern

45. <u>Contrarily to popular beliefs</u>, bats do not actually entangle themselves in the hair of humans on purpose.

a. Contrarily to popular beliefs
b. Contrary to popular belief
c. Contrary to popularity belief
d. Contrary to popular believing

46. Considering how long ago the Ancient Egyptians lived, it's amazing we know anything about them at all.

a. Considering how long ago the Ancient Egyptians lived, it's amazing
b. Consider how long the Ancient Egyptians lived, it's amazing
c. Considering for how long the Ancient Egyptians lived, its amazing
d. Considering, how long ago the Ancient Egyptians lived, its amazing

47. <u>Because technology has constantly changed</u>, those employed in the IT industry must learn new skills continuously.

a. Because technology has constantly changed
b. Because technology is constantly changing
c. Even though technology is changing
d. Despite the fact that technology has changed

48. <u>To mix, shade, and highlighting</u> are essential skills that every beginning artist must master.

a. To mix, shade, and highlighting
b. Mix, shade, and highlighting
c. To mixing, shading, and highlighting
d. Mixing, shading, and highlighting

49. The growing problem of resistance to antibiotics can be attributed, in part, <u>to the fact that they are prescribed unnecessarily</u>.

a. to the fact that they are prescribed unnecessarily
b. in the facts that they are prescribed unnecessarily
c. to the fact that they are prescribing unnecessarily
d. with the facts that they are being prescribed unnecessarily.

50. <u>A key challenges facing university graduates</u> searching for employment is that most have limited work experience.

a. A key challenges facing university graduates
b. Key challenge faced by university graduates
c. A key challenge facing university graduates
d. Key challenges facing university's graduates

51. Children who aren't nurtured during infancy are more likely to develop attachment disorders, <u>which can cause persisting and severely problems</u> later in life.

a. which can cause persisting and severely problems
b. that can cause persisting and severe problem
c. they can cause persistent and severe problem
d. which can cause persistent and severe problems

52. While speed is a measure of how fast an object is moving, velocity measures how fast an object is moving <u>and also indicates in what direction</u> it is traveling.

a. and also indicates in what direction
b. and only indicates in which direction
c. and also indicate in which directions
d. and only indicated in what direction

53. Many companies are now using social networking sites like Facebook and MySpace <u>to market there service and product.</u>

a. to market there service and product
b. to market their services and products
c. and market their service and products
d. which market their services and products

54. An autoclave is a tool used mainly in hospitals <u>to sterilizing surgical tools and hypodermic needles</u>.

a. to sterilizing surgical tools and hypodermic needles
b. for sterilize surgical tools and hypodermic needles
c. to sterilize surgical tools and hypodermic needles
d. for sterilizing the surgical tool and hypodermic needle

55. <u>The bizarre creatures known by electric eels</u> are capable of emitting an incredible 600 volts of electricity.

a. The bizarre creatures known by electric eels
b. A bizarre creature known as electric eels
c. The bizarre creatures known to electric eels
d. The bizarre creatures known as electric eels

56. <u>A key factor taken into account during city planning is</u> where major services and amenities will be located.

a. A key factor taken into account during city planning is
b. Key factors taken into account during city planning is
c. A key factor taking into account during city planning is
d. Key factors, taken into accounting during city planning are

57. Jupiter with its numerous moons, and Great Red Spot, has been studied extensively by astronomers.

a. Jupiter with its numerous moons, and Great Red Spot,
b. Jupiter with, its numerous moons and Great Red Spot,
c. Jupiter, with its numerous moons and Great Red Spot,
d. Jupiter with, its numerous moons, and Great Red Spot,

58. Many gardeners are now making their own backyard compost, which is not only cheap, but also helps to cut down on landfill waste.

a. which is not only cheap, but also helps to cut down on landfill waste
b. which is not only cheaper, but also cuts down on landfill's waste
c. which is, not only cheap, but also, helps to cut down on landfill waste
d. which is not only done cheaply, but is also cutting down on landfills wastes

59. <u>The growth of the security industry can be large attributable</u> to the fact that people are less trusting of others than they once were.

a. The growth of the security industry can be large attributable
b. The growing of the securities industry can be largely attributable
c. The growth on the security industry can be large attributed
d. The growth of the security industry can be largely attributed

60. Claude Monet was a famous painter <u>who's well-known painting includes</u> *San Giorgio Maggiore at Dusk* and *The Water Lily Pond*.

a. who's well-known painting includes
b. whose well-known painting including
c. whose well-known paintings include
d. who well-known paintings include

Answer Key and Explanations

Reading Comprehension

1. B: Paragraph 1 states the parents married before World War II, and everything that follows occurs after that.

2. C: The last sentence of the first paragraph identifies Nana as what the children called Marian's mother, who was therefore their grandmother. It also identifies Fluffy as the cat's name (B).

3. D: Sentence #6 of 8 in paragraph 2 states that Marian had contracted poison oak while petting the Irish setter, Katie, who had rubbed against Marian's bare legs.

4. A: Sentence #4 of paragraph 1 states that the couple lived with Marian's widowed mother. The last sentence of this paragraph also states that the children called Marian's mother Nana.

5. A: Sentence #3 of paragraph 1 says Bernard was in the Army. Sentence #4 refers to his tour of duty. This means the term a soldier serves in the military forces.

6. C: Paragraph 3 describes the family hearing Fluffy meow during dinner (B), but this was not how they discovered where he had been; it was by seeing him go back up the chimney where he had been hiding all along.

7. D: Paragraph 3 identifies the chimney as a cool place (B) to escape from all the commotion (C), so these are both correct. Cats generally tend to hide, but when frightened, not always (A).

8. C: Sentence 1 of paragraph 4 says cats hate changes in their environment (A), and identifies the noise and confusion of moving (B). The beginning of this sentence describes the cat's need for safety and seclusion/privacy (D). Paragraph 2 identifies a dog in the neighborhood (C), but not in the house; the passage states Fluffy was never outdoors. Fluffy could have smelled the dog's scent on Marian, who had petted her, and also from a distance; but considering the more direct factors of (A), (B), and (D), this is the *least* likely reason the cat found moving day traumatic.

9. C: The penultimate sentence of the final paragraph describes Fluffy doing (A), (B), and (D), but never mentions his climbing drapes in Lewis's room (C).

10. D: The main focus of the passage is how the family "lost" and then found their pet while moving. The other choices are all details included in the story rather than its main topic.

11. C: The earliest use of this title and lyric identified in this passage were by Al Dubin and Harry Warren in 1933. Billie Joe Armstrong (A) used it in 2004. Tony Bennett and Sting (B) recorded a duet covering the Dubin and Warren original in 2006. Gottfried Helnwein (D) gave his painting this title in 1984.

12. D: The passage states that Hopper named his famous painting *Nighthawks. Boulevard of Broken Dreams* (A) was the name of Gottfried Helnwein's painting, which was a parody of Hopper's *Nighthawks. American Idiot* (B) was the title of Green Day's 2004 album that included their original song, inspired by Helnwein's painting and also entitled *Boulevard of Broken Dreams. Strange Wine* (C) was the title of Harlan Ellison's 1978 collection of science fiction short stories, which included his story entitled *Boulevard of Broken Dreams.*

13. A: The passage says Constance Bennett sang this song in the 1934 movie. It says later that Tony Bennett and Sting (B) covered it in a duet in 2006. It identifies a different song with the same title being (written and) sung by Billie Joe (Armstrong) and Green Day (C) in 2004. And it states that Juan García Esquivel (D) recorded a song with this title in 1958.

14. B: The passage states that Hopper created his original painting using oils, and that Helnwein painted his parody of Hopper's work using watercolors.

15. D: The passage quotes these lyrics, identifying them as from the Green Day song written by Billie Joe Armstrong. The passage also quotes lyrics from the 1933 Dubin (A) and Warren (B) song, including "Here is where you'll always find me/Always walking up and down...." But the earlier song is never quoted to (and does not in fact) include "I walk alone, I walk alone" as Armstrong's song does. Constance Bennett (C) sang the older song in the movie *Moulin Rouge* but did not write it.

16. D: None of these celebrities are portrayed in Hopper's painting: the passage describes the four people in Hopper's painting as "anonymous." Dean (A), Presley (B), Monroe (C), and Humphrey Bogart are all depicted in Gottfried Helnwein's painting, a later parody of Hopper's work.

17. C: The passage indicates that Ellison published a short story with this title in 1978. It identifies Alexander's biography of Dean (A) as published in 1994. It states that Deitch's graphic novel (B) was published in 2002. And it identifies the E! TV network as airing a documentary series with this title (D) in 2007.

18. B: The passage reports that Green Day's song was inspired by Gottfried Helnwein's parody painting entitled *Boulevard of Broken Dreams.* The famous painting by Edward Hopper (A) was entitled *Nighthawks* and not named as an inspiration for Green Day's song. Neither is the 1933 song (C) of the same title, which was sung in the 1934 movie *Moulin Rouge* (D), also not Green Day's source.

19. A: This passage includes paintings, songs, albums, movies, books, and a TV series using the title. It identifies both single songs and albums (B); a science fiction book and a graphic novel (C); and a documentary series on TV (D).

20. A: The passage dates Helnwein's painting with the celebrities to 1984. It says the celebrities pictured had all died young between 1955 and 1977.* Thus they were not still alive [(C), (D)]. Since Helnwein made the painting seven years after the latest death and 29 years after the earliest one, they had not just recently died (B). *(James Dean died in 1955; Humphrey Bogart in 1957; Marilyn Monroe in 1962; and Elvis Presley in 1977.)

21. B: In describing the marketing of "sea monkeys," the author describes it as "creative genius" and attributes their popularity to the drawings and advertisements that appeared in comic books. It is reasonable to conclude that without the branding and (somewhat misleading) ads, they wouldn't have been as popular. Marketing them under the less exciting brand name "brine shrimp" likely wouldn't have resulted in as many sales.

22. C: Choice A is incorrect because the passage states that four-track tape and eight-track tape were similar in size. The cost of production is not mentioned, eliminating B as a possibility. D is incorrect because it was the eight-track tape that was included in these vehicles. C is correct because the passage states the eight-track tape could store and play twice as many songs.

23. B: The passage states that, "Often, the agoraphobic will view his home as the safest possible place to be, and he may even be reluctant to leave his house," making B the correct choice.

24. D: B and C are only briefly mentioned, allowing them to be eliminated as possibilities. Although the passage does discuss what could happen to two balls released at the top of a mountain, that is not the purpose of the passage, so A can be eliminated. The purpose is to show how small differences (in this case, two inches between two rubber balls) can have large effects. This is essentially what the butterfly effect is, and the purpose of the passage is to give an example to demonstrate this principle.

25. A: The passage discusses several problems that can occur with wells. Both of the problems mentioned are associated with wells that are too shallow; no problems associated with wells that are too deep are mentioned. Therefore, it seems safe to conclude that a deeper well would be more desirable than a shallow one.

26. C: A is mentioned only briefly in the passage. B and D are mentioned, but this information does not fit into the overall purpose of the passage, which is to discuss the different types of fats, both good and bad.

27. B: C and D are mentioned only briefly. Although the history of satire is discussed, most of the passage focuses on discussing the three major forms of satire that originated in Ancient Greece and Rome, making B the best choice.

28. A: B is incorrect because the passage states that happiness is expressed similarly by people all over the world. C is incorrect because the passage states that there are many emotions felt and expressed by people all over the world. D is incorrect because, although people may express acceptance differently, that is not sufficient to conclude it is not a natural emotion. A is correct. We can conclude that people can't always hide what they are feeling because of the statement in the passage that the facial expressions associated with emotions like fear are largely involuntary.

29. C: C is the correct answer because the passage mainly focuses on discussing the causes of heat island. A, B, and D are touched upon only in passing.

30. C: A and D are incorrect because the passage states that these are characteristics that marsupials and mammals share. B can be eliminated, because it is not mentioned in the passage. C is the correct choice, as "one thing that separates marsupials from mammals is that their young are born when they are not yet fully-developed" is stated in the passage.

31. B: Theists are the opposite of atheists, so the second sentence provides a contrast to the first.

32. C: The first sentence introduces the concept of home schooling. The second sentence states that one parent usually has to give up their job for home schooling to take place, which is a direct effect of the practice of home schooling.

33. D: The first sentence states that coffee is the most popular beverage. The second sentence directly contradicts it, stating that soda is the most popular. The second sentence contradicts the first.

34. B: A salamander's ability to grow a new tail is an example of the ability to replace severed body parts, which is known as regeneration. The second sentence provides an example of the concept explained in the first.

35. C: Both sentences give the same information, and nothing new is added. The second sentence restates the information from the first.

36. A: The second sentence tells how septic tanks can contribute to the problem of soil contamination. Both contamination and septic tanks are mentioned in the first sentence. Therefore, the second sentence expands on the first.

37. C: The first sentence states that the Richter Scale is the most commonly-used method to measure the strength of earthquakes. The second sentence states that other methods are used more frequently. Therefore, the second sentence contradicts the information in the first.

38. B: The first sentence introduces the concept of adaptation, which refers to an animal's ability to change in order to increase its chances of survival. A porcupine's quills allow it to defend itself against potential predators, thereby increasing its chances of survival. The second sentence provides an example of the concept presented in the first.

39. D: The first sentence states a problem: congestion due to excessive traffic. The second sentence offers a solution: carpooling can reduce the amount of traffic on roads, which could logically help ease congestion.

40. C: The first sentence describes how men make decisions. The second sentence describes the different process that is used by women to make decisions, which provides a contrast to the first.

Numerical Ability

1. D: This is a simple addition problem. Start with the ones column (on the right). Add the figures 6+1, 3+0, 2+3 to get the answer 537.

2. C: This is a simple addition problem with carrying. Start with the ones column and add 7+4, write down the 1 and add the 1 to the digits in the ten's column. Now add 0+6+1. Write down the 7. Now add 3+8 and write down the 1. Add the 1 to the thousand's column. Add 4+1+1 and write the 6 to get the answer 6171.

$$\begin{array}{r} 4307 \\ +\ 1864 \\ \hline \end{array} \qquad \begin{array}{r} {\scriptstyle +1} \\ 4307 \\ +\ 1864 \\ \hline 1 \end{array} \qquad \begin{array}{r} 4307 \\ +\ 1864 \\ \hline 71 \end{array} \qquad \begin{array}{r} {\scriptstyle +1} \\ 4307 \\ +\ 1864 \\ \hline 171 \end{array} \qquad \begin{array}{r} 4307 \\ +\ 1864 \\ \hline 6171 \end{array}$$

3. B: Substitute the given values for a and b and perform the required operations:

$$\begin{aligned} a^2 + 3ab - b^2 &= 3^2 + 3(3)(-2) - (-2)^2 \\ &= 9 - 18 - 4 \\ &= -13 \end{aligned}$$

4. A: This is a subtraction problem which involves borrowing to get the answer of 189.

$$\begin{array}{r} 356 \\ -\ 167 \\ \hline \end{array} \qquad \begin{array}{r} {\scriptstyle +10} \\ 346 \\ -\ 167 \\ \hline 9 \end{array} \qquad \begin{array}{r} {\scriptstyle +10+10} \\ 246 \\ -\ 167 \\ \hline 89 \end{array} \qquad \begin{array}{r} {\scriptstyle +10+10} \\ 246 \\ -\ 167 \\ \hline 189 \end{array}$$

5. B: This is a subtraction problem which also involves borrowing to get the answer of 1,819. In this case, it involves borrowing from zero, which just means that the zero needs to borrow from the next digit to become 10 and then it becomes 9 to lend to the original digit.

$$
\begin{array}{r} 5306 \\ -\ 3487 \\ \hline \end{array}
\quad
\begin{array}{r} {\scriptstyle +10} \\ 5206 \\ -\ 3487 \\ \hline \end{array}
\quad
\begin{array}{r} {\scriptstyle +9+10} \\ 5206 \\ -\ 3487 \\ \hline 9 \end{array}
\quad
\begin{array}{r} {\scriptstyle +9+10} \\ 5206 \\ -\ 3487 \\ \hline 19 \end{array}
\quad
\begin{array}{r} {\scriptstyle +10\ +9+10} \\ 4206 \\ -\ 3487 \\ \hline 819 \end{array}
\quad
\begin{array}{r} {\scriptstyle +10\ +9+10} \\ 4206 \\ -\ 3487 \\ \hline 1819 \end{array}
$$

6. C: This problem is solved by finding x in this equation: $\frac{32}{80} = \frac{x}{100}$.

7. A: This is a multiplication problem with 0. Start with the 7 in 17 and multiply it by each of the digits at the top 7×7. Write down the 9 and place the 4 in the ten's column. $7 \times 0 = 0$. Add the 4. $7 \times 7 = 49$. The top line will read 4949. Now multiply 1 by 7. Write down the 7. $1 \times 0 = 0$ and $1 \times 7 = 7$. The bottom line will read 707. Add these together with the 7 in the tens column and the answer will be 12,019.

$$
\begin{array}{r} 707 \\ \times\ \ 17 \\ \hline \end{array}
\quad
\begin{array}{r} {\scriptstyle +4} \\ 707 \\ \times\ \ 17 \\ \hline 4949 \end{array}
\quad
\begin{array}{r} 707 \\ \times\ \ 17 \\ \hline 4949 \\ 707\ \end{array}
\quad
\begin{array}{r} 707 \\ \times\ \ 17 \\ \hline 4949 \\ 707\ \\ \hline 12019 \end{array}
$$

8. A: This is a simple division problem. Divide the 7 into 9. It goes in 1 time. Write 1 above the 9 and subtract 7 from 9 to get 2. Bring down the 1 and place it beside the 2. Divide 7 into 21. It goes in 3 times. Divide 7 into 7. It goes 1 time.

$$
\begin{array}{r} 131 \\ 7\overline{)\,917} \\ \underline{7} \\ 21 \\ \underline{21} \\ 07 \\ \underline{07} \\ 0 \end{array}
$$

9. D: Recall that the general form of a quadratic expression is $ax^2 + bx + c$. A great way to factor quadratic expression like this, where $a = 1$ and all the answer choices are integer factors, would be to consider the factors of the last term, c. Specifically, any two factors of c that would add to b. Essentially: $f_1 \times f_2 = -12$ and $f_1 + f_2 = 1$. We can check the factors of -12:

f_1	f_2	$f_1 + f_2$
12	-1	11
6	-2	4
4	-3	1
3	-4	-1
2	-6	-4
1	-12	-11

From this it is clear that the only option that works is 4 and -3.

10. A: To change this fraction into a decimal, move the decimal to the right two places: 0.38.

11. C: This is a simple addition problem. Line up the decimals so that they are all in the same place in the equation, and see that there is a 6 by itself in the hundredths column. Then add the tenths column: 8+3to get 11. Write down the 1 and carry the 1. Add the ones column: 6+1 plus the carried 1. Write down 8. Then write down the 1.

12. A: A set of six numbers with an average of 4 must have a collective sum of 24. The two numbers that average 2 will add up to 4, so the remaining numbers must add up to 20. The average of these four numbers can be calculated: 20/4 = 5.

13. C: Recall that the thousandths place is the third digit to the right of a decimal:

0	.	3	8	**7**	4
ones	decimal	tenths	hundredths	**thousandths**	ten thousandths

14. A: This is a subtraction problem with decimals. Be sure to line up the decimals.

$$\begin{array}{r} 0.58 \\ -\ 0.39 \\ \hline \end{array} \qquad \begin{array}{r} {\scriptstyle +10} \\ 0.48 \\ -\ 0.39 \\ \hline 9 \end{array} \qquad \begin{array}{r} {\scriptstyle +10} \\ 0.48 \\ -\ 0.39 \\ \hline 0.19 \end{array}$$

15. D: This is multiplication with decimals. It is often easiest to perform the multiplication on the numbers without the decimals and then figure out where to put the decimal in the final result. To do this, convert the decimals to fractions and then multiply:

$$0.25 \times 0.03 = \frac{25}{100} \times \frac{3}{100} = \frac{25 \times 3}{100 \times 100} = \frac{25 \times 3}{10000} \qquad \begin{array}{r} {\scriptstyle +1} \\ 25 \\ \times\ \ 3 \\ \hline 75 \end{array} \qquad \frac{75}{10000} = 0.0075$$

16. A: To add fractions, ensure that the denominator (the number on the bottom) is the same. Since it is not, change them both to 56ths. 1/8 equals 7/56. 3/7 equals 24/56. Now add the whole numbers: $3 + 6 = 9$ and the fractions 31/56.

$$3\frac{1}{8} + 6 + \frac{3}{7} = (3 + 6) + \left(\frac{1}{8} + \frac{3}{7}\right) = (3 + 6) + \left(\frac{7}{56} + \frac{24}{56}\right) = (9) + \left(\frac{31}{56}\right) = 9\frac{31}{56}$$

17. C: To subtract fractions, ensure that the denominator (the number on the bottom) is the same. Since it is not, change them both to 14ths. $1/7 = 2/14$; $1/2 = 7/14$. The equation now looks like this: $4\frac{2}{14} - 2\frac{7}{14}$. Change the 4 to 3 and add 14 to the numerator (the top number) so that the fractions can be subtracted. The equation now looks like this: $3\frac{16}{14} - 2\frac{7}{14} = 1\frac{9}{14}$.

18. A: To multiply mixed numbers, first create improper fractions. Multiply the whole number by the denominator, then add the numerator. $1\frac{1}{4}$ becomes $\frac{5}{4}$; $3\frac{2}{5}$ becomes $\frac{17}{5}$; $1\frac{2}{3}$ becomes $\frac{5}{3}$. Now, multiply all the numerators together and then all the denominators together:

$$\frac{5}{4} \times \frac{17}{5} \times \frac{5}{3} = \frac{5 \times 17 \times \cancel{5}}{4 \times \cancel{5} \times 3} = \frac{85}{12} = 7\frac{1}{12}$$

19. C: For this problem there are 3 inches in each segment, 12 inches in a foot, and 3 feet in a yard. Set up a conversion problem and simplify:

$$4.5\ \cancel{\text{yd}} \times \frac{3\ \cancel{\text{ft}}}{1\ \cancel{\text{yd}}} \times \frac{12\ \cancel{\text{in}}}{1\ \cancel{\text{ft}}} \times \frac{1\ \text{segment}}{3\ \cancel{\text{in}}} = 4.5 \times 12\ \text{segments} = 54\ \text{segments}$$

20. C: Divide the numerator and denominator by 14.

21. D: Recall that 'percent' means per 100. So, the fraction $\frac{36}{100}$ is the same as 36 per 100 or 36%.

22. C: 40% can be thought of as 40 per hundred. Since there are 9 hundreds in 900, then there will be 9 forties in 40% of 900: $9 \times 40 = 360$.

23. A: If it takes 3 people 3 1/3 days to do the job, then it would take one person 10 days: $3 \times 3\frac{1}{3} = 10$. Thus, it would take 2 people 5 days, and one day of work for two people would complete 1/5 of the job.

24. A: Divide 40 by 8 to get 5. Multiply 5 by 3 to get 15.

$$\frac{3}{8} \times 40 = 3 \times \frac{40}{8} = 3 \times 5 = 15$$

25. B: Rewrite the problem as $\frac{6}{100} \times 25$. Since $4 \times 25 = 100$:

$$\frac{6}{4 \times \cancel{25}} \times \cancel{25} = \frac{6}{4} = \frac{3}{2} = 1.5$$

26. D: Divide 4 by 16 (not 16 by 4) to get 0.25. Then move the decimal two places to the right to find the percentage.

27. C: Since 4 is the same as 2^2, $4^6 = 2^{12}$. When dividing exponents with the same base, simply subtract the exponent in the denominator from the exponent in the numerator.

$$2^{12} \div 2^8 = 2^{12-8} = 2^4 = 16$$

28. D: To solve, rewrite the percentage as a fraction: $\frac{30}{100}$. Then reduce the fraction: $\frac{3}{10}$.

29. C: To change a percent to a decimal, remove the percent sign and move the decimal two spaces to the left.

$$37\% \rightarrow 0.37$$

30. A: To solve, add $6a$ and $2a$, then subtract $4a$.

$$-4a + 6a + 2a = -4a + 8a = 4a$$

31. B: The order of operations dictates that addition and subtraction be computed as each appears, from left to right, in the expression. Thus, the expression can first be rewritten as $18 + 7 + 5 + 11$. The expression can next be rewritten as $25 + 5 + 11$. Finally, the expression can be rewritten as $30 + 11$, which equals 41.

32. D: The following expression can be used to represent the problem: $5.50 - (3.25 + 2.00) + 3.50$. The order of operations requires that the computation within parentheses be handled first. Thus, the expression can be rewritten as $5.50 - 5.25 + 3.50$. The expression can next be rewritten as $0.25 + 3.50$, which equals 3.75. So, Luis had \$3.75 in his wallet at the end of the day.

33. A: The order of operations dictates that any computations within parentheses be first calculated. Thus, the expression can be rewritten as $\frac{1}{3} + \frac{2}{15} - \frac{2}{15}$. The additive inverse property reveals that the last two terms in the expression sum to 0, leaving $\frac{1}{3}$ as the answer.

34. E: The problem requires 13.71 feet of wire be subtracted from the total number of feet purchased, or 14.5 feet. The difference is 0.79. John had 0.79 feet of wire left over after fixing the lamp.

35. D: A non-member must pay $\$12 \times 7$, or \$84, for all 7 CDs. A member pays \$24 for all 7 CDs. Thus, Maria saves $\$84 - \$24$, or \$60, by joining the club.

36. A: The difference is equal to 7,576,000. This number can be written in scientific notation by moving the decimal point behind the 7, in the millions place, and counting the number of digits to the right of the decimal point. The number, written in scientific notation, is 7.576×10^6.

37. D: The inequality can be rewritten as $3 < \sqrt{x} < 5$. Each term in the inequality can be squared, in order to eliminate the square root symbol. Thus, the inequality can be written as $(3)^2 < \left(\sqrt{x}\right)^2 < (5)^2$, or $9 < x < 25$.

38. D: The rule of exponents states that $x^{\frac{a}{b}} = \sqrt[b]{x^a}$. Thus, $\sqrt[3]{27} = 27^{\frac{1}{3}}$, or 3. Thus, the product can be written as 3×3, or 9.

39. B: A proportion in the form $\frac{a}{b} = \frac{c}{d}$ can be rewritten as $ad = bc$. Thus, the given proportion can be solved for x as follows: $11x = 49$, where $x = \frac{49}{11}$.

40. C: The problem can be represented by the proportion, $\frac{12}{\$48.75} = \frac{13}{x}$. The solution is equal to $\frac{\$48.75 \times 13}{12}$, or $\frac{13}{12} \times \$48.75$.

41. E: The number of people who passed the exam is equal to 0.80×55, or 44. Since 55 people took the exam, the number of people who failed the exam is equal to $55 - 44$, or 11.

42. C: In order to convert the fraction, $\frac{3}{4}$, into a percent, the fraction must first be converted to a decimal. In order to do so, the denominator of the fraction must be divided into its numerator; $3 \div 4 = 0.75$. The decimal, 0.75, can be converted to a percent by moving the decimal point two places to the right. Thus, 75% of the participants crossed the finish line in less than 3 hours.

43. C: Since the first three SAT scores summed to 1,900, the following equation can be used to find the score on the fourth exam: $\frac{1{,}900 + x}{4} = 650$. The equation can be solved for x by multiplying both sides of the equation by 4. Doing so gives: $1{,}900 + x = 2{,}600$. Subtracting 1,900 from both sides of the equation gives $x = 700$. Thus, he scored 700 on his fourth SAT exam.

44. C: The average time can be represented by the expression, $\frac{3}{4}(16) + \frac{1}{4}(12)$, which equals the sum of 12 and 3, or 15. Thus, the average time overall was 15 seconds.

45. B: Since she made \$21 in commissions during the first 3 hours, the following equation can be used to find the dollar amount she must make during the fourth hour: $\frac{\$21+x}{4} = \$8$. The equation can be solved for x by multiplying both sides of the equation by 4. Doing so gives: $\$21 + x = \$32$. Subtracting \$21 from both sides of the equation gives $x = \$11$. Thus, she must make \$11, in commissions, during the fourth hour, in order to average \$8 per hour for the full four hours.

46. C: When the numerator and denominator of a fraction are divided or multiplied by the same number, the quotient or product is equivalent to the original fraction. In this case, the numerator and denominator of 6/12 can be divided by two, giving 3/6.

47. D: 675 × 7 = 4,725

48. C: 5,465 + 394 = 5,859

This is closest to 6000 (C).

49. C: Multiply 1/6 by 2 to get a common denominator.

1/6 × 2 = 2/12

Then calculate 11/12 – 2/12 = 9/12

Reduce this fraction by dividing both numerator and denominator by 3.

(9 ÷ 3) / (12 ÷ 3) = 3/4

50. B: 743 – 87 = 656

Language Ability

1. A: When it is said that someone is generous, it usually means they are giving and unselfish.

2. C: When something is described as challenging, it usually means that it is difficult or demanding.

3. B: A teacher provides instruction and information to an individual or group of individuals. An instructor functions in the same capacity, that is, in the practice of teaching.

4. D: When something is concluded, it means that it is finished or completed.

5. A: A residence is a place where a person lives; the term is often used to refer to someone's home.

6. C: To say something was done instantly means that it was done immediately and without hesitation.

7. C: Something that is described as gigantic is extremely large, or huge, in size.

8. A: Something that is costly is expensive. It costs a lot of money.

9. D: An opportunity is a chance to do something. For example, saying someone was given the *opportunity* to go to school or saying somebody was given the *chance* to go to school conveys the same meaning.

10. B: A response is also commonly known as an answer. A response to a question carries the same meaning as an answer to a question.

11. C: To say that something is done frequently implies that it is done regularly or often.

12. A: Something that is being observed is being watched. Binoculars are used to see things more clearly, so it makes sense that the man would be observing or watching eagles with binoculars.

13. D: Saying that somebody purchased something and saying they bought something conveys the same meaning.

14. D: The word difficulty implies hardship. When it is said that somebody is having difficulties with another person or thing, it usually means they are experiencing problems.

15. A: Entire is an amount. It usually means the whole amount. For example, if someone says they ate an entire apple, it is the same as saying they ate a whole apple.

16. C: To say something is superior to something else usually implies that it is better.

17. B: A remark is a spoken statement, also commonly known as a comment. To say somebody made a remark conveys the same meaning as saying they made a comment.

18. C: When a selection is being made, it involves making a choice between several options. Selecting something is the same as choosing something.

19. A: To commence something is to begin or start something.

20. B: When something is done swiftly, it means that it is done fast or quickly.

21. A: separate

22. B: nuclear

23. C: familiar

24. A: sacrilegious

25. C: agitated

26. B: oriented

27. C: indispensable

28. A: similar

29. B: attitude

30. B: abbreviate

31. A: absorb

32. C: accumulate

33. C: aerial

34. A: comedian

35. B: asphalt

36. B: forcible

37. C: anecdote

38. A: flexible

39. A: defendant

40. C: plaintiff

41. B: The phrase *to have extinction* in choice A is grammatically incorrect. In choice C, *causes* is plural, and so the word should be *exist* rather than *exists*. D is not the best choice because it is somewhat awkward. B sounds the best and is also grammatically correct.

42. C: C is the best answer because it indicates a contrast and is grammatically correct.

43. A: A is the best answer because it denotes the party to whom companies are offering tech support and because the verb *are* agrees with the noun *customers*.

44. D: D is the best choice. The phrases *high-fat diets* and *excessive amounts of television* agree with each other because they are both plural. The word *is* refers to *the fact that*, so these also agree with each other.

45. B: This is a well-known phrase meaning *despite what most people believe*. The word *contrarily* in choice A makes it incorrect. *Popularity* in choice C is out of place, and *believing* in choice D is incorrect.

46. A: B implies the Egyptians had long life spans, which doesn't make sense in the context of the sentence. C uses *its* instead of the grammatically correct *it's*, while D has misplaced commas and also uses *its*. A indicates the Egyptians lived a long time ago, and the correct form of *it's* is used.

47. B: The sentence describes a cause/effect relationship, so *because* is the correct way to begin the sentence. Choice A implies that technology changed in the past, which does not make sense in the context of the sentence. B indicates a cause/effect relationship, and states that technology is continuously changing, which is why IT professionals must continuously learn new skills.

48. D: Choice D is correct because the three verbs are in the same form. Choices A and B use different verb forms. Choice C is grammatically incorrect because of the *to* that is used to begin the sentence.

49. A: Saying that something can be *attributed to* something else is grammatically correct, which eliminates choices B and D. C is incorrect because *they* refers to antibiotics, so the sentence is essentially stating that antibiotics are prescribing. Inanimate objects are incapable of doing this, which makes the sentence incorrect. Choice A states that antibiotics are prescribed, indicating someone else is doing the prescribing, which makes it the correct choice.

50. C: A is incorrect because *a* and *challenges* do not agree. B is incorrect because *key challenge* must be prefaced by *A* D is incorrect because of the misplaced apostrophe, and also because the sentence only identifies one challenge, meaning the plural, *key challenges*, is incorrect.

51. D: Answer choice A is incorrect because *severely* is an adverb and not an adjective. B and C are incorrect because *problem* instead of the grammatically correct *problems* is used. D uses the correct, plural form *problems* and uses adjectives to describe the problems.

52. A: The sentence implies that *velocity* is used to indicate more than one value, which eliminates B and D. The phrase refers to velocity, which is singular, but the construction of choice C would correctly refer to a plural noun. Choice A agrees with the singular, noun and the *and* indicates that velocity is used to indicate more than one value.

53. B: Answer choice B uses the grammatically correct *their* instead of *there*. The *to* indicates the companies are using these sites for something, and *services* and *products* agree with each other because they are both plural.

54. C: Answer choice C states that an autoclave is a tool used *to sterilize*. A and B, which begin with *to sterilizing* and *for sterilize*, are not grammatically correct. D indicates that the machine is used to sterilize a single tool and needle, which does not make sense in the context of the sentence.

55. D: Answer choices A and C are incorrect because they imply that the bizarre creatures are something other than electric eels. The *a* in choice B does not agree with the plural *electric eels*. Choice D is best because it is grammatically correct and identifies electric eels as the bizarre creatures being discussed in the sentence.

56. A: Answer choice B is incorrect because the plural *key factors* and the singular *is* do not agree. The *taking* in choice C makes it incorrect. Choice D has a misplaced comma. Choice A makes sense and the singular *a key factor* and *is* agree with each other.

57. C: Choice C is the only choice that has correctly placed commas. The *numerous moons* and the *Great Red Spot* both refer to the planet Jupiter, which is maintained in answer choice C.

58. A: Answer choice B is incorrect because of the misplaced apostrophe. C has two unnecessary commas. Answer choice D is too wordy, and *landfills wastes* sounds quite awkward. Answer choice A is succinct, the comma is in the correct place, and it expresses the information is a clear way that is not awkward.

59. D: Answer choices A and C are incorrect because *large* is used in front of *attributable* and *attributed*. Both of these phrases are grammatically incorrect. B describes *the growing of the securities industry*, which is quite awkward. D is the best choice because it refers to *the growth of the security industry* and uses the phrase *largely attributed*, which is grammatically correct.

60. C: The correct way to refer to a person, in this case Monet, is through the use of the pronoun *whose*, which eliminates A and D. Two paintings are identified, so the plural form must be used, eliminating choice B. Choice C uses *whose* and *paintings*, indicating there is more than one, making it the correct choice.

How to Overcome Test Anxiety

Just the thought of taking a test is enough to make most people a little nervous. A test is an important event that can have a long-term impact on your future, so it's important to take it seriously and it's natural to feel anxious about performing well. But just because anxiety is normal, that doesn't mean that it's helpful in test taking, or that you should simply accept it as part of your life. Anxiety can have a variety of effects. These effects can be mild, like making you feel slightly nervous, or severe, like blocking your ability to focus or remember even a simple detail.

If you experience test anxiety—whether severe or mild—it's important to know how to beat it. To discover this, first you need to understand what causes test anxiety.

Causes of Test Anxiety

While we often think of anxiety as an uncontrollable emotional state, it can actually be caused by simple, practical things. One of the most common causes of test anxiety is that a person does not feel adequately prepared for their test. This feeling can be the result of many different issues such as poor study habits or lack of organization, but the most common culprit is time management. Starting to study too late, failing to organize your study time to cover all of the material, or being distracted while you study will mean that you're not well prepared for the test. This may lead to cramming the night before, which will cause you to be physically and mentally exhausted for the test. Poor time management also contributes to feelings of stress, fear, and hopelessness as you realize you are not well prepared but don't know what to do about it.

Other times, test anxiety is not related to your preparation for the test but comes from unresolved fear. This may be a past failure on a test, or poor performance on tests in general. It may come from comparing yourself to others who seem to be performing better or from the stress of living up to expectations. Anxiety may be driven by fears of the future—how failure on this test would affect your educational and career goals. These fears are often completely irrational, but they can still negatively impact your test performance.

Elements of Test Anxiety

As mentioned earlier, test anxiety is considered to be an emotional state, but it has physical and mental components as well. Sometimes you may not even realize that you are suffering from test anxiety until you notice the physical symptoms. These can include trembling hands, rapid heartbeat, sweating, nausea, and tense muscles. Extreme anxiety may lead to fainting or vomiting. Obviously, any of these symptoms can have a negative impact on testing. It is important to recognize them as soon as they begin to occur so that you can address the problem before it damages your performance.

The mental components of test anxiety include trouble focusing and inability to remember learned information. During a test, your mind is on high alert, which can help you recall information and stay focused for an extended period of time. However, anxiety interferes with your mind's natural processes, causing you to blank out, even on the questions you know well. The strain of testing during anxiety makes it difficult to stay focused, especially on a test that may take several hours. Extreme anxiety can take a huge mental toll, making it difficult not only to recall test information but even to understand the test questions or pull your thoughts together.

Effects of Test Anxiety

Test anxiety is like a disease—if left untreated, it will get progressively worse. Anxiety leads to poor performance, and this reinforces the feelings of fear and failure, which in turn lead to poor performances on subsequent tests. It can grow from a mild nervousness to a crippling condition. If allowed to progress, test anxiety can have a big impact on your schooling, and consequently on your future.

Test anxiety can spread to other parts of your life. Anxiety on tests can become anxiety in any stressful situation, and blanking on a test can turn into panicking in a job situation. But fortunately, you don't have to let anxiety rule your testing and determine your grades. There are a number of relatively simple steps you can take to move past anxiety and function normally on a test and in the rest of life.

Physical Steps for Beating Test Anxiety

While test anxiety is a serious problem, the good news is that it can be overcome. It doesn't have to control your ability to think and remember information. While it may take time, you can begin taking steps today to beat anxiety.

Just as your first hint that you may be struggling with anxiety comes from the physical symptoms, the first step to treating it is also physical. Rest is crucial for having a clear, strong mind. If you are tired, it is much easier to give in to anxiety. But if you establish good sleep habits, your body and mind will be ready to perform optimally, without the strain of exhaustion. Additionally, sleeping well helps you to retain information better, so you're more likely to recall the answers when you see the test questions.

Getting good sleep means more than going to bed on time. It's important to allow your brain time to relax. Take study breaks from time to time so it doesn't get overworked, and don't study right before bed. Take time to rest your mind before trying to rest your body, or you may find it difficult to fall asleep.

Along with sleep, other aspects of physical health are important in preparing for a test. Good nutrition is vital for good brain function. Sugary foods and drinks may give a burst of energy but this burst is followed by a crash, both physically and emotionally. Instead, fuel your body with protein and vitamin-rich foods.

Also, drink plenty of water. Dehydration can lead to headaches and exhaustion, especially if your brain is already under stress from the rigors of the test. Particularly if your test is a long one, drink water during the breaks. And if possible, take an energy-boosting snack to eat between sections.

Along with sleep and diet, a third important part of physical health is exercise. Maintaining a steady workout schedule is helpful, but even taking 5-minute study breaks to walk can help get your blood pumping faster and clear your head. Exercise also releases endorphins, which contribute to a positive feeling and can help combat test anxiety.

When you nurture your physical health, you are also contributing to your mental health. If your body is healthy, your mind is much more likely to be healthy as well. So take time to rest, nourish your body with healthy food and water, and get moving as much as possible. Taking these physical steps will make you stronger and more able to take the mental steps necessary to overcome test anxiety.

Mental Steps for Beating Test Anxiety

Working on the mental side of test anxiety can be more challenging, but as with the physical side, there are clear steps you can take to overcome it. As mentioned earlier, test anxiety often stems from lack of preparation, so the obvious solution is to prepare for the test. Effective studying may be the most important weapon you have for beating test anxiety, but you can and should employ several other mental tools to combat fear.

First, boost your confidence by reminding yourself of past success—tests or projects that you aced. If you're putting as much effort into preparing for this test as you did for those, there's no reason you should expect to fail here. Work hard to prepare; then trust your preparation.

Second, surround yourself with encouraging people. It can be helpful to find a study group, but be sure that the people you're around will encourage a positive attitude. If you spend time with others who are anxious or cynical, this will only contribute to your own anxiety. Look for others who are motivated to study hard from a desire to succeed, not from a fear of failure.

Third, reward yourself. A test is physically and mentally tiring, even without anxiety, and it can be helpful to have something to look forward to. Plan an activity following the test, regardless of the outcome, such as going to a movie or getting ice cream.

When you are taking the test, if you find yourself beginning to feel anxious, remind yourself that you know the material. Visualize successfully completing the test. Then take a few deep, relaxing breaths and return to it. Work through the questions carefully but with confidence, knowing that you are capable of succeeding.

Developing a healthy mental approach to test taking will also aid in other areas of life. Test anxiety affects more than just the actual test—it can be damaging to your mental health and even contribute to depression. It's important to beat test anxiety before it becomes a problem for more than testing.

Study Strategy

Being prepared for the test is necessary to combat anxiety, but what does being prepared look like? You may study for hours on end and still not feel prepared. What you need is a strategy for test prep. The next few pages outline our recommended steps to help you plan out and conquer the challenge of preparation.

Step 1: Scope Out the Test

Learn everything you can about the format (multiple choice, essay, etc.) and what will be on the test. Gather any study materials, course outlines, or sample exams that may be available. Not only will this help you to prepare, but knowing what to expect can help to alleviate test anxiety.

Step 2: Map Out the Material

Look through the textbook or study guide and make note of how many chapters or sections it has. Then divide these over the time you have. For example, if a book has 15 chapters and you have five days to study, you need to cover three chapters each day. Even better, if you have the time, leave an extra day at the end for overall review after you have gone through the material in depth.

If time is limited, you may need to prioritize the material. Look through it and make note of which sections you think you already have a good grasp on, and which need review. While you are studying, skim quickly through the familiar sections and take more time on the challenging parts.

Write out your plan so you don't get lost as you go. Having a written plan also helps you feel more in control of the study, so anxiety is less likely to arise from feeling overwhelmed at the amount to cover.

Step 3: Gather Your Tools

Decide what study method works best for you. Do you prefer to highlight in the book as you study and then go back over the highlighted portions? Or do you type out notes of the important information? Or is it helpful to make flashcards that you can carry with you? Assemble the pens, index cards, highlighters, post-it notes, and any other materials you may need so you won't be distracted by getting up to find things while you study.

If you're having a hard time retaining the information or organizing your notes, experiment with different methods. For example, try color-coding by subject with colored pens, highlighters, or post-it notes. If you learn better by hearing, try recording yourself reading your notes so you can listen while in the car, working out, or simply sitting at your desk. Ask a friend to quiz you from your flashcards, or try teaching someone the material to solidify it in your mind.

Step 4: Create Your Environment

It's important to avoid distractions while you study. This includes both the obvious distractions like visitors and the subtle distractions like an uncomfortable chair (or a too-comfortable couch that makes you want to fall asleep). Set up the best study environment possible: good lighting and a comfortable work area. If background music helps you focus, you may want to turn it on, but otherwise keep the room quiet. If you are using a computer to take notes, be sure you don't have any other windows open, especially applications like social media, games, or anything else that could distract you. Silence your phone and turn off notifications. Be sure to keep water close by so you stay hydrated while you study (but avoid unhealthy drinks and snacks).

Also, take into account the best time of day to study. Are you freshest first thing in the morning? Try to set aside some time then to work through the material. Is your mind clearer in the afternoon or evening? Schedule your study session then. Another method is to study at the same time of day that you will take the test, so that your brain gets used to working on the material at that time and will be ready to focus at test time.

Step 5: Study!

Once you have done all the study preparation, it's time to settle into the actual studying. Sit down, take a few moments to settle your mind so you can focus, and begin to follow your study plan. Don't give in to distractions or let yourself procrastinate. This is your time to prepare so you'll be ready to fearlessly approach the test. Make the most of the time and stay focused.

Of course, you don't want to burn out. If you study too long you may find that you're not retaining the information very well. Take regular study breaks. For example, taking five minutes out of every hour to walk briskly, breathing deeply and swinging your arms, can help your mind stay fresh.

As you get to the end of each chapter or section, it's a good idea to do a quick review. Remind yourself of what you learned and work on any difficult parts. When you feel that you've mastered the material, move on to the next part. At the end of your study session, briefly skim through your notes again.

But while review is helpful, cramming last minute is NOT. If at all possible, work ahead so that you won't need to fit all your study into the last day. Cramming overloads your brain with more information than it can process and retain, and your tired mind may struggle to recall even previously learned information when it is overwhelmed with last-minute study. Also, the urgent nature of cramming and the stress placed on your brain contribute to anxiety. You'll be more likely to go to the test feeling unprepared and having trouble thinking clearly.

So don't cram, and don't stay up late before the test, even just to review your notes at a leisurely pace. Your brain needs rest more than it needs to go over the information again. In fact, plan to finish your studies by noon or early afternoon the day before the test. Give your brain the rest of the day to relax or focus on other things, and get a good night's sleep. Then you will be fresh for the test and better able to recall what you've studied.

Step 6: Take a Practice Test

Many courses offer sample tests, either online or in the study materials. This is an excellent resource to check whether you have mastered the material, as well as to prepare for the test format and environment.

Check the test format ahead of time: the number of questions, the type (multiple choice, free response, etc.), and the time limit. Then create a plan for working through them. For example, if you have 30 minutes to take a 60-question test, your limit is 30 seconds per question. Spend less time on the questions you know well so that you can take more time on the difficult ones.

If you have time to take several practice tests, take the first one open book, with no time limit. Work through the questions at your own pace and make sure you fully understand them. Gradually work up to taking a test under test conditions: sit at a desk with all study materials put away and set a timer. Pace yourself to make sure you finish the test with time to spare and go back to check your answers if you have time.

After each test, check your answers. On the questions you missed, be sure you understand why you missed them. Did you misread the question (tests can use tricky wording)? Did you forget the information? Or was it something you hadn't learned? Go back and study any shaky areas that the practice tests reveal.

Taking these tests not only helps with your grade, but also aids in combating test anxiety. If you're already used to the test conditions, you're less likely to worry about it, and working through tests until you're scoring well gives you a confidence boost. Go through the practice tests until you feel comfortable, and then you can go into the test knowing that you're ready for it.

Test Tips

On test day, you should be confident, knowing that you've prepared well and are ready to answer the questions. But aside from preparation, there are several test day strategies you can employ to maximize your performance.

First, as stated before, get a good night's sleep the night before the test (and for several nights before that, if possible). Go into the test with a fresh, alert mind rather than staying up late to study.

Try not to change too much about your normal routine on the day of the test. It's important to eat a nutritious breakfast, but if you normally don't eat breakfast at all, consider eating just a protein bar. If you're a coffee drinker, go ahead and have your normal coffee. Just make sure you time it so that the caffeine doesn't wear off right in the middle of your test. Avoid sugary beverages, and drink enough water to stay hydrated but not so much that you need a restroom break 10 minutes into the test. If your test isn't first thing in the morning, consider going for a walk or doing a light workout before the test to get your blood flowing.

Allow yourself enough time to get ready, and leave for the test with plenty of time to spare so you won't have the anxiety of scrambling to arrive in time. Another reason to be early is to select a good seat. It's helpful to sit away from doors and windows, which can be distracting. Find a good seat, get out your supplies, and settle your mind before the test begins.

When the test begins, start by going over the instructions carefully, even if you already know what to expect. Make sure you avoid any careless mistakes by following the directions.

Then begin working through the questions, pacing yourself as you've practiced. If you're not sure on an answer, don't spend too much time on it, and don't let it shake your confidence. Either skip it and come back later, or eliminate as many wrong answers as possible and guess among the remaining ones. Don't dwell on these questions as you continue—put them out of your mind and focus on what lies ahead.

Be sure to read all of the answer choices, even if you're sure the first one is the right answer. Sometimes you'll find a better one if you keep reading. But don't second-guess yourself if you do immediately know the answer. Your gut instinct is usually right. Don't let test anxiety rob you of the information you know.

If you have time at the end of the test (and if the test format allows), go back and review your answers. Be cautious about changing any, since your first instinct tends to be correct, but make sure you didn't misread any of the questions or accidentally mark the wrong answer choice. Look over any you skipped and make an educated guess.

At the end, leave the test feeling confident. You've done your best, so don't waste time worrying about your performance or wishing you could change anything. Instead, celebrate the successful completion of this test. And finally, use this test to learn how to deal with anxiety even better next time.

Review Video: Test Anxiety
Visit mometrix.com/academy and enter code: 100340

Important Qualification

Not all anxiety is created equal. If your test anxiety is causing major issues in your life beyond the classroom or testing center, or if you are experiencing troubling physical symptoms related to your anxiety, it may be a sign of a serious physiological or psychological condition. If this sounds like your situation, we strongly encourage you to seek professional help.

Online Resources

Due to our efforts to try to keep this book to a manageable length, we've created a link that will give you access to all of your online resources:

mometrix.com/resources719/pnat

It's Your Moment, Let's Celebrate It!

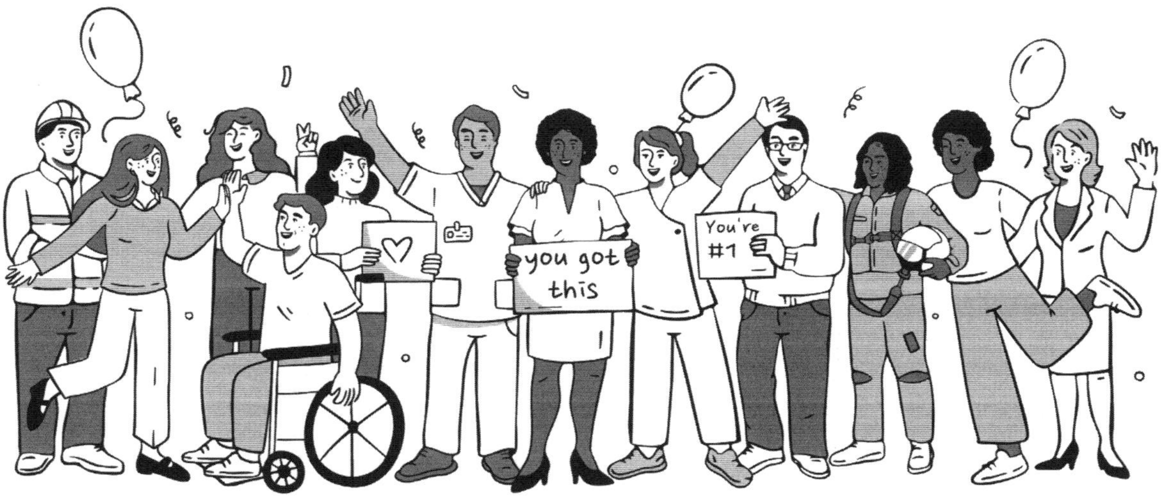

Share your story @mometrixtestpreparation